The 30 Day Body Hack

Elaine DiRico

With

Chef Billie Dixon III

ISBN: 1502597896
ISBN-13: 9781502597892

DEDICATION

For Billie Dixon III, and Bruce Thompson, my Fellow Food Ninjas

Yvonne Magee, and Dr. Ellen Lewis my sisters and willing taste testers

Deborah Samson, my friend and editor

And

Dr. Abbas Quatab, and Dr. Marlene Merritt who continue to inspire me

Introduction

'All you have to do is write one true sentence.'

~Hemingway

A good beginning. I have always loved this quote, and it has helped me sort through a lot of the chaff in my life. One would think it would be easy, but I find it to be challenging, and soul revealing. It is what I want this book to be: a series of true sentences.

Most of us have spent a lot of our lives working, being in relationships, cleaning and cooking, and hopefully having some fun as well. I worked two jobs for a lot of my adult life, and raised kids, taking care of a home and a husband, and was also in school for a lot of those years. I was blessed with good health, and enjoyed my life hugely. But in my fifties, I had a health challenge, like so many of us do. I was lucky, in that it wasn't life threatening, but it landed me in a wheelchair for a couple of years. It also gave me a lot of time to read and think and reflect on my life.

Imagine that every person gets one car to last their entire life. Only one car ever. Maintenance would be done religiously! From the beginning, we would want to keep the car running optimally and would be very careful with it. Yet, knowing we will only be issued one body, at least this time around, we don't lavish the same sort of care on our bodies that we would on that car. In fact, most of us metaphorically drive as hard and fast as we can until the car simply stops running. This is what I called a 'health challenge.'

For this to change, we need a new paradigm, similar to the 'One Car per Life' model. We see health not as something to nourish, support and optimize, but rather as not being sick. And thanks to Big

1

2Pharmaceutical Companies, if we feel unwell, there is always a pill… and then another pill for the first pill's side effects and a pill for those side effects. Surely no one can watch a pharmaceutical commercial with a straight face any more! We look to the medical community to fix what ails us. But there is one fallacy in this that brings it all down like a house of cards: by treating a symptom, you are not addressing the underlying cause, and a new symptom will pop up somewhere like the 'Whack-A-Mole' game at the carnival until the underlying cause is resolved.

I am a Nutritional Therapist. I see the world through the context of food as medicine. I have always been enthralled with food, cooking and everything surrounding food. I have owned a restaurant, written cookbooks, cooked in logging and archeology camps, as well as cooked the majority of my family's meals for decades. I am happiest in the kitchen. When I was finally released from rehabilitating my injury (2 years and 8 surgeries later) I was even heavier than when I was first injured, and had learned a lot about depending on the kindness of others. I still had too much pain; I was depressed and fat, and saw my doctor, precisely as instructed by all those commercials. His response was to suggest pain killers and antidepressants.

Well, that didn't happen. I started reading; I found a doctor of Chinese Medicine/ Nutritionist who started me on a new path. Since I was effectively retired, back to school I went. I can't tell you what a pleasure it has been to study, without the pressure of grades and time, and to study something I have always loved: food. My doctor, Marlene Merritt, has been my inspiration and my mentor, my friend…. and she also saved my life.

While I began this book as a diary, documenting a thirty day detox program, it has quickly morphed into an account of how my ideas about living an optimal life have changed over the last five years. It is still tied to the form of a diary, but you are also going to get a lot of opinion, stories and hopefully a few laughs along the way. I am not a doctor, and though it sounds like I am disparaging the medical profession, I don't intend to. As much as I love Marlene, if I break a leg, I want to see a surgeon, not an acupuncturist! But until recently, with the creation of Integrative Medicine, most of what lay outside the practice of medicine was considered 'alternative' and pooh-poohed by the same medical and pharmaceutical professionals who would lose money if these other options were found to work. . Even nutrition was seen as frivolous. And that makes sense if you are getting rich selling crappy food.

Recently I was speaking to a group of first year medical students at Texas A&M. One question was: 'How can we, as doctors, help our patients with their nutrition?' I have thought a lot about the idea, and my answer now would be: 'Western medicine is predicated on the idea that a body is broken, and needs outside intervention to fix it. Nutrition and other alternative health care disciplines are based on the idea that a body is self-healing, much more than we have imagined, and that given the proper fuel, can heal itself. While these are not completely incompatible ideas, I believe having a Nutritional Therapist in your office is the solution. There is so much that you, as medical students, have to learn, without adding an entire other discipline. Bring a good solid person in and refer your clients. Let them make money for you and let them give you more information about your patients than you would have otherwise.'

This is the paradigm change I have made, which has transformed my life. I know with certainty that my body is doing everything it can to keep me happy and healthy, and that the best investment of time, energy and money that I can make is giving my body everything it needs to be optimally healthy. This includes a good orthopedic surgeon when I break it. It is not only the best one I have, it is the only one. This is my story. It is an account of the many things I have tried over the course of a long life, and what my experience has been. I hope that it can give you some ideas, support and thoughts about your life, and what you can make of it. No matter where your ambitions lie, starting with optimal health is the best thing you can do to maximize the odds of success.

Phase One:

In December of 2012, I was in Houston, fulfilling my CEU's requirement with a class on Detoxification taught by Dr. Abbas Qatab. Over the years, I had become somewhat jaded on the idea of detoxing, and I was not terribly excited about this speaker, whom I knew nothing about. The Western Medicine party line on the subject seems to be: 'We are self-cleaning, just like ovens.' The photograph in the brochure showed an attractive, but unsmiling man, in a suit and tie. It was looking like a long weekend...

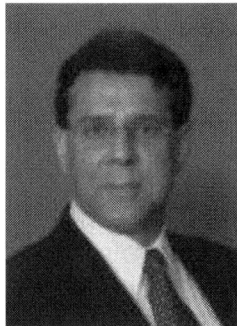

And it turned out to be a remarkable weekend. Dr. Qatab has more letters after his name than in his name, including a Ph.D. in both Ayurvedic Medicine and Chinese Medicine, he is and an MD, and also a Chiropractor. He is one of those remarkable people who can think outside of several boxes at the same time. It was a wonderful weekend, and transformed my ideas about detoxification, as well as renewing my faith in my body's innate wisdom and capacity to heal.

The idea that we are self-cleaning is true, but it doesn't take into account that for the first two hundred million years of life on this earth, there were not *nearly* as many toxins as there are today. There was stress of course, often in the form of accidents, starvation, and sudden death. But the amount of chemical toxins that we eat and drink and breathe has increased geometrically over the last fifty years with no end in sight. The filtration system that we had evolved centered around our digestion and liver, was probably up to most anything we could throw at it. It is different today. According to Dr. Mark Hyman, fatty liver, which simply means 'overwhelmed liver', is the most common disease in the United States, and 80,000,000 Americans suffer from it. [1] While it is called 'fatty liver' the issue is not fat, but rather sugar. Like a goose or duck being fed grains to create fois gras, it is fructose and other sugars that are killing us. According to Hyman, he is seeing 12 year old boys who have been drinking soda all of their lives on lists for liver transplants. Most people who have this going on don't even know it. The key to healing is changing our diet. The first phase of this program is designed to mega dose your entire system with enzymes to jump start elimination.

In the back of this book, you will find a list of foods that are recommended that you eat while doing this program. It is also available on my web site, where you can print it and tape it to the refrigerator. I have done the entire thirty day cleanse three times, and I am just starting my fourth round as I write this. It is not a weight loss diet, although you may lose weight. It is a regimen that will change how you eat, hopefully permanently. There will be very little coming into your kitchen in a box. From the first day, you will eliminate the foods and drinks from your life that are known to be the most damaging and reactive. In a month, as you gradually add them back in, you will have a chance to see how your body reacts to them when it isn't used to them. This phase can be very enlightening. And as you move to a diet of whole REAL foods, things your great grandparents would recognize, you are likely to find that you react even more to things like Diet Coke, Oreos and other refined foods. You may also discover that the foods you eat the most are also the ones you react to the most.

Use organic, fresh foods as much as possible. You are detoxifying to remove the chemicals and poisons from your body; it is important to avoid adding more toxins. Organic labeling only means that it was grown organically: once it is harvested, it may no longer be regulated. This and freshness are good reasons to get to know a farmer. The old adage that every dollar you spend is a vote applies here. Supporting sustainable, organic farms is a vote for a better future. Regardless of the source, wash your produce. I use cold water, and a splash of vinegar. As a general rule, the good germs love acid and the bad germs hate it.

Another consideration is the healing crisis. As your body works to move toxins, you might experience any of a number of effects. While conventional western medical care might try to suppress these symptoms, it is important to remember that they are an indication that your body is healing itself. Headaches, mild nausea, a rash, aches, or fatigue are some of the more common effects. They may come on suddenly, and may last a few hours, or rarely, a few days. The operative word here is healing, and once the crisis is past, know that you will feel much better than before the symptoms developed. In fact, the stronger the crisis, the deeper the cleanse is thought to be. Relax, call your healthcare provider if you feel the need for support, and know that you are giving your body a chance to reverse a long, gradual disease process. If you should become too uncomfortable, ask your provider to change your supplement schedule. This may extend the period of Phase One.

Minimizing stress in every way possible is a good practice. Plan a bedtime, and make every effort to keep it. Shut down all of your 'screens' a full hour before going to bed. This means computers, e-book readers, televisions and notebooks. All of these emit light that can be very disruptive to your Circadian rhythms. An actual book or magazine can be a relaxing change. An Epsom salt soaking bath is another way to facilitate sleep- the magnesium in the warm water is a muscle relaxant and the heat allows your body temperature to drop when you get out of the tub. Lower body temperatures encourage good sleep. A drop of lavender oil also relaxes. If you can schedule 9 hours every night to stay in bed whether you sleep or not, you may find that alarm clocks are not necessary, and that your quality of sleep improves. It is only thirty days, and sleep is a vital part of health. If you have a history of sleep disorders, schedule a sleep study with your ENT. Lack of sleep contributes to every aspect of ill health, including cardiac issues, diabetes and obesity.

Are you ready? This is not about self-denial. It is about self discovery. Since you are motivated and in change mode, I am going to suggest some other things you might try just to see if they have a place in your life and if they can make you happier or healthier or both.

1.   http://drhyman.com/blog/2013/09/26/fatty-liver-90-million-americans/

Phase One, Day 1

Here we go! There is a list of questions in the appendix, as well as on my web site, that you can download and print every night. These will be very useful when you finish your detox, to look back and relive the experience. It is easy to forget and change and edit our experiences as we distance from them. I want you to keep it fresh. While a health problem is almost always the incentive for doing a detox, remembering how good you felt, how clear headed and happy you were, and especially, how surprisingly easy the whole process was can be the support you need to make a detox a regular part of your health regimen. This is also a great way to get into the habit of journaling.

What you can take away from this simple 30 day program:

- renewed energy, vigor and health
- improved digestion
- improved absorption of nutrients
- a new appreciation for 'real food'
- a better connection with what your body needs to function optimally
- better sleep, better sex
- better management of your stressors
- knowledge how to cook simple, healthy meals
- a working knowledge of how much the health of our country has been compromised by the Big Farm and Big Pharm corporations, and why keeping us ill makes them richer and richer

Not a bad deal for one month.

You will begin your Detoxification by taking large doses of enzymes three times a day, to begin 'moving things along.' This whole exercise is about what you put into your body, how it passes through and how you can make this as comfortable, efficient and beneficial as possible. Most people know that food goes in your mouth, out your other end, and something obscure happens in the interim. (To understand what actually happens, you might google 'digestion videos.') Because the SAD (Standard American Diet) has, in the last few decades, included more and more 'processed foods' and less 'Real Food,' our digestive systems need new methods of support.

Processing a food can mean anything: cooking, grinding, sterilizing and adding color, preservatives, flavors and other chemicals. The primary purpose is to create a longer shelf life, so the naturally occurring enzymes that would aid digestion are suppressed. Because sugar can inhibit bacterial growth, it is often found in processed foods, usually in the form of High Fructose Corn Syrup, or HFCS. Instead of eating fresh fruits and vegetables that will enhance our own enzymes, we are eating foods that need less work to digest, like HFCS or other foods which are indigestible, like hydrogenated fats and rancid, cheap oils that are most often used in processed foods. This is why the fresher the food is, and the less processed, refined foods you eat, the more nutrition you will absorb. Of course, these refined foods are also low in fiber, and are almost like baby food. They are digested very quickly, and, since they are extremely low in nutrition, we remain hungry. A brilliant plan by the food manufacturers to keep us eating, and in fact to make high refined sugar/ cheap fat/ high refined salt based foods addictive.[1]

Most of us don't eat fresh, high quality, nutritionally dense foods, so Phase One introduces a variety of enzymes, in quantity, to begin clearing things and get digestion revved up to eliminate the accumulated gunk. These are food based, some fermented, as well as some animal sourced enzymes. Beets are an important addition as well, to thin bile. When you take your first dose, you may feel odd. On rare occasions, nausea occurs, but usually there is little more than perhaps a little gurgle. These symptoms pass quickly, as your body accustoms itself to the new regime, but if you are uncomfortable at all, halve the dosage and take a few more days in Phase One to build up to the full dose. And as always, have your healthcare professional on speed dial!

Breakfast. We have been taught by everyone from Kellogg's to Kashi (and Kellogg's bought Kashi in 2000) that grains are the perfect breakfast. Certainly it is the perfect breakfast if you own Kellogg's stock, or Nabisco, General Mills and on and on. For the sake of your nutrition, though, it is not worth much. Grains are very different now than they were even 20 years ago, and they are grown on exhausted, mono-cropped farms whose mineral and vitality deficient soil was depleted decades ago. Add in GMOs, lectins, and the fact that we simply haven't been eating grains long enough to have adapted well to them, and they are clearly not the nutrient rich foods that we are looking for. In a few days, the problem will be solved with the whey·shakes, and a smoothie is a fine way to begin the day. The traditional carb rich breakfast gives us a quick lift, but quickly leaves us hungry. What you are doing when you eat is building a metabolic fire. Carbohydrates, like kindling, light quickly and burn fast, but needs constant replenishment. Protein and fats are like burning a nice sturdy hardwood log. They burn slowly and steadily and for much longer. Refined

9

starches and sugars, like pancakes with HFCS based maple syrup, or biscuits or cereal burn like lighter fluid...

One of the best lifetime habits to adopt for daily detoxification is to drink a liter of water with the juice of a lemon first thing upon waking. I fill a bottle before going to bed every night, which makes it more difficult to forget. You will be avoiding caffeine for the next month and this habit helps ease cravings. Your body has spent the night doing a lot of housekeeping chores, cleaning things out, and in the process, dehydrating. There is nothing better than a nice, slightly acidic, delicious flush to get everything ready for the day. This can go down quickly, as the purpose is to wash things out. Imagine cleaning and sweeping your house all night, then, instead of getting the debris into the trash, you leave it in a pile by the door. Of course it will get re-absorbed! The rest of the day, sipping water regularly to rehydrate until you have a total of three or four liters for the day is perfect, although in the summer, especially in the South, more is better.

Finally: I have always found it easy to get lost in work and sit for far too long at once. My solution of late has been to set a timer for an hour, get up, get a big glass of water, walk around or hop on the stationary bike, get some blood flow back to my brain, stretch, and in general behave as my dogs do. This actually increases significantly the amount of work I can get done as well as the quality of the work.

Phase One, Day 2

Congratulations! You have already survived the toughest day. It seems like a lot of changes to make, and it will be well worth it. At the same time, you are educating yourself on everything about your relationship with food. There will be some things that you miss more than others, and make sure to put that in your journal. Thirty days is a long enough period to break some habits and when you finish your program, you can choose which ones to let back into your life. There will be surprises, there may be some struggles, but thousands of people have gone through this process, and you can do it as well. From moment to moment, the choice is always yours.

Here is a visual that I use a lot when I teach classes on nutrition and change.

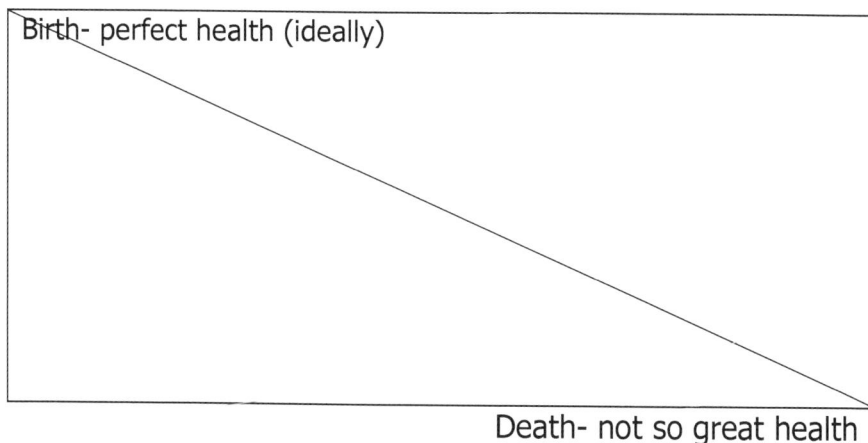

Birth- perfect health (ideally)

Death- not so great health

Every decision you make is going to put you above or below that line. Make enough right decisions, and approaching eighty can feel pretty good. But this really means *every* decision. "One Diet Coke won't hurt" moves you below the line. No one is perfect, and a perfect life would be unbearable. Just know that every decision counts and every decision is entirely up to you. {{Kicking aside soapbox}}

Once we try to take control of our food and food sources, we learn that planning is the key to success. Our species is hardwired to eat whenever we get the chance. Without that imperative, we wouldn't have survived. But until my generation, the Baby Boomers, we simply didn't have that many opportunities to eat. My mother grew up during the Dust Bowl on a ranch in Southwestern

11

Oklahoma, and had a lot of firsthand experience with hunger. Yet all of my grandparents lived into their nineties. It isn't hunger that shortens most of our life spans, but the opposite. Eating too much nutritionally empty food is another form of hunger, and because we aren't getting the elements we need, we keep eating, keep eating, keep eating.

We have learned, largely through advertising, that food is entertainment, and we look forward to it as a break in the day. I am asking you to start looking at food differently. Think of it as two sorts of food. First is food as fuel. This is the 'real food' I have mentioned. It is as fresh and clean and as full of vitality as we can make it. Organic, and delicious, may be an acquired taste, but acquiring it can save our lives. It can also make every day of our lives better and more enjoyable. The second food is feasting food. It can be anything, and its purpose is to connect with loved ones, celebrate and enjoy. This element is as important as the quality of the food, I believe; call it emotional and spiritual nutrition. No one wants to skip a piece of birthday cake at a toddler's party, or a glass or two or three of champagne at a wedding. Thanksgiving, at a table surrounded by loved ones is not a time to whip up a spinach and pear smoothie. But we can choose the healthy, life giving foods most of the time so that when we have an opportunity to feast and enjoy life and sit and relax and talk and laugh around a table, we have the capacity to do so without impacting our health too badly. To me, this is as much the purpose of making healthy choices as anything else.

Of course, the trick becomes a matter of pacing. If we believed the world we see in the media, every day is a feast, and we will be slender and healthy and beautiful regardless. This has not been my experience. Every meal, once you learn more about what your body needs and enjoys, can be a delicious, renewing time, but the feasts are just that- occasional or even rare treats, that we relish and make the most of.

Lunch, for most of us, is on the fly. It is important to have options, which means packing a lunch. Insulated lunchboxes, reusable ice blocks and a little planning make this easy and affordable. It sometimes seems like eating real food is expensive, but keep in mind that restaurants, even fast food restaurants, can be expensive too. The SAD (Standard American Diet) is unsustainably cheap because it is made largely from subsidized crops like corn, wheat, soybeans and rice. Instead of comparing your food bill to the cost of three happy meals a day, compare it to my sister in Scotland, who spends around thirty percent of the family income on food. If you lived in Brazil, you would spend about a quarter of your income to eat, and Indonesia, Egypt and most of Africa spends almost half of their money on food. In the US, it is less than seven percent.[1] And those fast food meals made from subsidized grains, raised on unsustainable corporate farms? Not as cheap as they seem, since the subsidies, most of which are paid to corporations, come out of our tax dollars.[2]

Here is what works best for me: I go to the Farmer's Markets once a week, usually Saturday. This is my favorite thing to do all week, so I set out to enjoy it. Here in Austin, we have a lot of food trailers who strive to use the local, organic and sustainable foods available. You will often find several at the Farmer's Markets. When I am eating with restrictions, I take advantage of their work. The relationships I have built with the farmers and purveyors are invaluable. They are often the people who picked the food earlier that morning, gathered the eggs; they know what is good today and what will be ready next week. I go with a general idea of what I need, but it is important also to be flexible, to take advantage of the season. This is often a couple of hours of very enjoyable hunting and gathering, but if it is not your thing, take a friend, or organize a group and send a different person each week to buy for everyone.

I like to get my proteins at Farmer's Markets as well, but this is not so easy. Once you find a butcher and a fishmonger, treasure the relationship. Austin is blessed with several options, and I have even split a side of beef with friends. Costco has begun getting some excellent organic chicken from the Coleman Ranch. You will find that the meat has more texture and more flavor than the factory raised birds. They get to walk around and make friends and such, and I prefer to vote with my dollars by buying them. Yes, they are more than a dollar a pound, but as Joe Salatin has said, 'You think eating organic food is expensive? Have you priced cancer lately?' The more you know about your food sources, the better your meals will be. Another way to consider it is the nutritional value, then subtract the toxins, and

The same goes for eggs. I like to meet my hens, if I can, and know that they have a good life, roaming and eating all kinds of bugs and greens and such while they harvest that Vitamin D from the sun and pack it into my eggs for me. Jeremiah Cunningham (www.coyotecreekfarm.org/eggs/) raises some lovely hens, and keeps them away from soy, which suits me fine. At $6 or so a dozen, they seem pricey, but at a dollar for a meal's worth of excellent protein, they are a steal. I keep a half dozen of them hard boiled in the refrigerator.

I spend a lot of Saturday doing food prep, but the time is well spent. Dinner rarely takes more than fifteen minutes of actual work to get to the table. Salad greens are washed, dried and put into a pillowcase. I wash enough for a couple of salads a day for the week. If you are buying packaged greens, yes they have been washed, probably repeatedly. I wash them again, with a splash of white vinegar in the water for the bad bugs like *e. coli.* I am happiest when I wash the

13

lettuces from the farmers markets and there are a couple of bugs and some sand at the bottom of the sink. Good enough for bugs to eat means good enough for me to eat. Spinach and collards and kale get the same treatment, different pillowcase.

Vegetables get washed, and stored. I don't cut them up until I am ready to use them, as they will lose nutrition as soon as the cells are exposed. Tomatoes on the counter, stem end down, everything else in bins. Fruit is mostly on the counter, but I wash it as well. An inordinate amount of food related illnesses come from cantaloupe of all things. They need a rich soil, which in most countries means manure. The rinds are right on the soil, and it is the rinds that we handle, then passing the pathogens to the fruit as we cut it up, believing that it was locked safely inside the fruit. Ooops.

No grains mean no bread to store. Proteins are always the longest prep time, so I often cook several meals worth of chicken and portion them out, bag them and freeze them. If I find grass fed hamburger meat at a good price, I get some to freeze, but cook off a couple of pounds, with onions and garlic and perhaps some green chilies; portion, pack and freeze. You get the idea.

And regarding bread. I know lunch without a sandwich seems impossible to most of us. But you may be very surprised by what a month without grains does for your overall health. One solution is butter lettuce. Everything that I want on my sandwich, plus maybe a few more vegetables, goes in a jar, and some butter lettuce leaves get packed separately. Roll the sandwich makings up like a burrito, and enjoy. Alternatively, anything that you would eat on bread goes just fine on a salad. By eliminating the 200 or so empty calories from the bread, you get to enjoy more of the good stuff.

Packing a salad is easy too. A quart mason jar, with the homemade dressing (recipes follow) in first, then protein, vegetables and finally greens. Pack a fork and plate, and when the lunch bell sounds, find a tree, crank up your IPod, take the deep breaths, be grateful and enjoy.

Basic Vinaigrette

The traditional ratio is 3 parts of oil (check the list of allowable oils) and one part of acid- this can be citrus juice, vinegar, or a combination. This may be a little to 'bright' for you, so find the ratio that works, get an empty bottle and using nail polish or an indelible marker, measure the two ingredients in and mark the levels. Anything extra, like a dab of mustard, chopped herbs, salt and pepper, gets added last and shaken in. Keep in the fridge.

14

"Ranch Dressing" is problematic. It is ubiquitous, and I have known kiddos who refused to eat a vegetable without it. The base is dairy (a no-no for now) and mayonnaise (commercial versions are made with a nightmare ingredient list of oils and additives, and few of us make our own.) The commercial version is very high in sugar, and in fact, for those kids, was a major source of the refined carbohydrates in their diets. If you really want to make a similar dressing, use chopped fresh herbs, such as chives, parsley, dill and some salt and pepper. For the base, find a coconut or almond yogurt and whisk in some good oil. If you like olive oil's flavor, great, use that. If it is too strong, avocado oil or a nut oil like walnut is milder. Store in the refrigerator.

This should get you some ideas on what you can pack. Even if I am just heading to the post office, I try to have a meal in the cooler, just in case. Like going to the store for 'just one thing' a one stop errand just never seems to work out. I have also started carrying my water in a quart Mason jar, packed with ice against an Austin summer. A hole drilled in the lid accommodates a straw if you like, and I have just read too much about plastics and the dangers to be comfortable with a plastic container for something I drink all day. I am also too cheap to buy a $30 thermos and leave it somewhere. Still haven't found a solution for my zip-lock baggie addiction, but life is really all about the negotiations, isn't it?

1) Source: USDA

2) http://articles.mercola.com/sites/articles/archive/2012/02/27/us-farm-subsidies-absurd.aspx

Phase One, Day Three

Life will be getting a little easier by now. The schedule is getting familiar, and so there is a little less to think about. The enzymes are busy doing their work, and maybe you aren't feeling quite as deprived with the diet regimen. The lemon water upon rising has probably changed your bathroom experience somewhat and the enzymes will be doing their part. All of this is part of the process, but certainly, if you have questions, call your health care provider.

Meals are settling in to a routine. Once you have learned what foods are supportive of the process and what foods can interfere with it, you will doubtless be making good choices, and very likely are feeling better already. The foods that are off the list of accepted foods can be problematic and are the ones that many people are sensitive to. Remember, this doesn't just mean an allergy- it can be an intolerance, or an acquired sensitivity, but eating these foods can put more stress on your digestive and immune system. As you gradually add them back in, post-detox, you will be able to tell readily which ones may not be your best choices.

The foods on the accepted list are the opposite. They support both digestion and detoxification, and allow your body to take a break, relax and heal. Green herbs like parsley, cilantro, basil and scallions are especially fine for healing and cleaning your body, so use them with abandon.

Most often, a health problem moves a person to consider a detox program, and I suspect you are no exception. By eliminating the stress of a heavy toxic load, you may be able to short circuit a self perpetuating inflammatory cycle. This course is longer, but less arduous than many. It also gives you room to address other stresses in your life. Because your body will be quite busy, it is a good time to look at where you are spending your precious energy. By choosing the very best foods, if only for this month, you can get a much clearer look at how diet can impact every aspect of your life. The questionnaire you fill out daily (and you ARE doing that right?), and perhaps a journal as well, will offer a clear reminder of how it feels to run on excellent fuel. You have noticed that there are questions about emotions in the mix. For me, this is the greatest benefit of a detox. Once some of the sludge is gone, and great food is coming on board, my body can delight in making the brain chemicals that disappear quickly when I am overstressed. Enjoy this part, and write a lot about it. These notes can be invaluable to get us back to clean eating rather than the old habits.

Clean protein is one of the most challenging foods to find. By now, you know my prejudices for Farmer's Markets, but it is also worthwhile seeking out farms that raise their animals carefully and humanely. Don't trust that because you found the beef at a health food store, it is necessarily free of GMOs, antibiotics and hormones. (I am looking at you, John Mackey...) Ask questions, call corporate offices, and if necessary, climb the managerial labyrinth to get answers. If a market knows that their customers are aware, involved, concerned, and most of all questioning, they will want to have answers that will make those customers happy and keep their business. If you are a regular at a particular store, you will be noticed. Be sure to offer support and compliments as often as possible, which will give your questions more importance and credibility. Again- use your dollars to support the food that you deserve. I believe this has as much or more impact as your votes.

Coleman Ranch, www.colemannatural.com is one of the largest producers of high quality, sustainably raised meats and poultry and their products are widely available. Their web site lists stores, and everything I have been able to find out about the company seems to support the quality of their meat. They are headquartered in Golden, Colorado, so for most of us, can't really qualify as local.

US Wellness meats is a mail order company. Family run, it is located in Canton, Missouri, and has very high quality, well cared for animals. If grocery shopping is a challenge for you, making a month's worth of menus, placing an order and filling your freezer might just be your best stress management technique. Since your meat arrives frozen, shipping can get pricey, but a large order can spread that out a bit. See if friends and family would like to place their orders at the same time, and save more.

If you are in Austin, check out my beloved Salt and Time. This new artisanal butcher shop and salumeria at 1912 East 7th St is foodie heaven. Like many high quality foods, the prices seem higher, but in fact, you find that its greater nutrition makes smaller portions quite satisfying. How's that for a win-win? When I have found myself away from my kitchen, the plates at their restaurant have been life savers. If you have trouble getting over a craving for fast food burgers, their products may do the trick. Once you are reminded how clean, well raised meat can taste, it is hard to stomach what passes for meat from corporate 'restaurants.' www.saltandtime.com.

Dai Due, at 2406 Manor Rd. here in Austin, roughly across from the Vortex Theater, is another amazing source for high quality meats. They specialize in game, and also produce beautiful bone broth and soups. Breakfast, lunch and dinner service is available, and the cooking and butchering happens just on the other side of the counter. www.daidue.com.

When you reduce refined carbohydrates, cut back on fats to spare your liver, and also reduce your serving size of protein, your vegetable intake is going to skyrocket. This is a fine thing. The statistics say that we were gradually increasing our consumption of vegetables until 2005, and the amount consumed per capita has dropped every year since. The average American is said to eat two servings a day. Although French fries are included, I think ketchup is left out of the veggie count, possibly because few people actually consume the required ½ cup to count as a serving. 'Food deserts' as portrayed in the documentary 'A Place at the Table' are responsible for some of this change, but the revenue generators in food production are not the row farmers. As happens with corporations, when the bottom line becomes more important than actual human beings, there will not be a good result.

Right now, you are in a perfect position to make some changes. Your palate is clearing, you are feeling better, and the whole idea of transformation has a lot of appeal. It is a fine time to explore some new recipes, new ideas and new foods! Commercial chips are an amazingly complex chemistry project, with layers of salt,chemicals, cheap fats, flavorings and sugar carefully engineered to make sure you can't eat just one. Mindlessly consuming a huge bag of Doritos is the easiest thing in the world to do. But there are options. Most root vegetables, like beets, carrots, and even potatoes can be made into quite serviceable chips. Zucchini is another option. Play with it...

Sweet Potato Chips
1 lb. Peeled sweet potato

1 Tbsp. Nutritional Yeast (optional for umami)

1 Tbsp. Olive Oil or Coconut Oil

Redmond Sea Salt or Pink Salt to taste

Pre-heat oven to 400 degrees. Thinly slice potatoes using a mandolin or a knife. The thinner the cut, the crispier the chip will be when done. Line a baking sheet with parchment paper and arrange the potatoes in a single layer. These guys need space to crisp up! Lightly brush the chips with oil/salt/yeast mixture, and bake for 20 minutes, until the edges curl and turn crispy. If they need more time, don't sweat it! Turn your oven down to 350°, and keep a close eye on them until the edges begin to brown. Cool on a rack to let them crisp while you start your next batch.

Phase One Day Four

You are probably wondering if today is the day you start Phase Two. Trust yourself, and the wisdom of your body. Are you well-adjusted to the enzymes you have been taking? Still a little gurgling in the tummy area? Nothing terrible will happen if you start the next phase today, nor will anything go wrong if you wait another day or two, so just relax. I always find that the shakes simplify my life, so as soon as my digestion feels settled in, I move on.

The shakes are simple- 8 to 12 ounces of liquid plus 2 scoops of Nutriclear and 1 scoop of Biotics Research Whey Isolate. The liquid can be water, so packing a to-go jar with the dry ingredients is simple. Shaker jars are widely available, and a water fountain is all you need. Of course, a base like coconut milk or almond milk is tasty, and a few berries can be delicious, but even the most basic shake is a nourishing meal substitute.

The purpose of Phase Two, and the shakes in particular is 'Metabolic Clearing.' This simply means supporting the body's processes for clearing toxins, such as environmental, dietary and anything that we take in that isn't of use or isn't recognized by our bodies. Toxins from medications, alcohol, food additives, our water, insecticides and even the potentially harmful waste that our intestinal bacteria excrete accumulate and cause inflammation. The more we are storing, the more energy and health is wasted that we could be putting to better use. This is the real work phase of the thirty days. The first few days are devoted to easing your body into readiness to get rid of waste, and then the last week is rebuilding, rather like spring cleaning. First you move the furniture out of the room, then you spend the most time actually cleaning and scrubbing everything, and finally, you get to move everything back in and enjoy.

You will also be taking the Bio-Detox Packs. These have a complete and balanced array of nutrients, and are convenient. It couldn't be easier. They will help you feel well while you let your body do its work, and also supply support for the elimination process. They will replace any supplements that you are already taking, but not medications.

You're set. Whether you move to the second step today is up to you, but keep this an enjoyable process. Evidence is building about the importance of gratitude as a stress reduction method and cardiac healer. I find that, as my head clears, it is remarkably easy to be grateful, and like the self-perpetuating inflammatory response, gratitude can be self-perpetuating. The whole food system in our country is remarkable, and to live in a time and a place where there are so many choices is an enormous gift. It is easy to romanticize the past, and imagine gathering eggs before school so that Mama could whip me up breakfast on the wood burning stove, and I could scamper off down a shaded country lane. Reality had a lot more to do with grueling work, manure, and long hours to put food on the table. The real blessing is to have the best of both, and access to the knowledge so we can make good choices about our health.

Good choices are the real key. Because the shakes have such complete nourishment, I find I rarely get hungry. I eat a big raw salad sometime during the day, and because I am lucky enough to love to cook, we usually have one 'traditional' meal. I find it easy to make a good quantity of protein, serve it once for a meal, and then scavenge it for salads and wraps during the week. Especially in the heat of summer, if I am turning on the oven, it is going to be full, so if I roast a chicken, I am putting a few vegetables to roast as well. I still try for a no-meat Monday, so let's call this:

Tuesday Night Dinner

1 large organic chicken*

Olive oil

1 organic lemon

6 or more garlic cloves, whole

Fresh herbs if you like. Parsley, sage rosemary and thyme are nice

Salt and pepper

Preheat your oven to 500°. There is a bit of controversy about rinsing chickens. One school holds that you are getting rid of the bacteria, the other believes that you are spreading it. I usually go with my whim. If there is a lot of water gathered in the packaging, I am more likely to rinse, but do keep it confined to a sink and then scrub the sink down with vinegar water. (Good bacteria love acid; the bad boys hate it…)

I have a vertical roaster for chickens that I love. It stores flat, is made by Norpro, and is available online. The third time you roast your own chicken instead of buying a rotisserie chicken, it pays for itself. When you take your chicken out of the fridge, let it come up to room temperature (about ½ an hour) to ensure even cooking. I give the bird a good rub with the olive oil, salt and pepper more than I think I need to, roll the herbs and garlic (no need to peel) together and push into the cavity. Then I cut the lemon in half and squeeze some juice over the chicken and put them cut side inward, into the cavity. Easy enough to sit her up on the vertical roaster, but if you are using a roasting pan, use the cut lemon and perhaps one more to sit the bird on to keep her off the surface of the pan. Ten minutes at high heat with the exhaust fan on starts a nice brown, crisp skin while you cut the vegetables.

Tomatoes, halved if they are large

Onions, peeled and quartered

Mushrooms

Fennel bulbs

Sweet potatoes, cut in ½" slices

Summer squash, in half inch slices

Lemons, halved

Whole heads of garlic

You can use your imagination here, and add carrots, turnips, sweet potato wedges, even cauliflower and broccoli. I line the rimmed baking sheets with parchment paper or foil, as the juices often get very sticky. Toss the vegetables with olive oil, salt and pepper, and dried herbs if you like. A splash of balsamic or sherry vinegar is always welcome. Drop the temperature in the oven to 325° and slide the vegetables in beside the chicken. They may cook at varying speeds, so keep an eye on them while you make a salad. Flip them with tongs or a spatula and if they seem to be cooking unevenly, rotate the pans. Take them out as they finish cooking. If you want them crisp, cool them on a rack, but if you want to preserve the juices, put them in a bowl and cover. This can be a side dish tonight, ratatouille tomorrow and soup the next day. The chicken will need about 25 minutes, depending on her size, to get the breast meat to 160 °. Let her rest on a platter for 10 minutes before your slice into the meat, or all the wonderful juice will run out. The temperature will also come up a few degrees as she rests. Discard the lemon and herbs; they have given up their soul for the gravy.

*Bigger chickens roast better, have better flavor and provide more leftovers.

If you are feeling ambitious, you can brine the chicken to make it more tender and juicy. In a large bowl, mix a handful of sea salt in warm water until it dissolves. Add a Tablespoon of honey (facilitates browning,) and whatever flavors you like. Add the chicken, and fill with cold water just to cover. Refrigerate or add ice and leave out on the counter. Either way, a half hour before you are planning to put her in the oven, drain the brine and pat her dry. Leave her out to warm up to room temperature for a bit so that she will cook evenly.

Alternatively, the day before you plan to roast the chicken, take her out of the wrappings, and salt her heavily all over.   Michael Polan suggests using three times the amount of salt that you think you need, which I find to be about right. In this preparation, it is providing a mechanical and chemical process more than a flavoring. Wrap the bird up again in cling wrap, and refrigerate.

After dinner, spend a couple of minutes deboning the roasted chicken and saving in individual servings in the freezer. Mark and date them- I always plan to remember what they are and never do, leading to an annual freezer purge that is daunting. And save your bones! One of the great joys of an organic chicken is making bone broth. Freeze them if you don't have enough to make a batch yet.

Phase One, Day Five

If you have already moved to Phase Two, go ahead and read through this anyway, just to get some more ideas.

I hope you are starting to feel a little smug. I know of nothing that is harder to do than change your eating habits. By choosing to eliminate many of the foods that are frequent troublemakers, you are, no doubt, beginning to have a sense of how much better you can feel every day. The food industry has done a fine job of convincing us that we deserve intensely flavored, entertaining, cheap food several times a day, yet we spend much less of our income on food in this country than anywhere else in the world and much more on 'health care.' This is a complete reversal from just a few years ago. As Hippocrates and many others have said since: 'Let food be your medicine.'

Geek Alert: I tend to get a little OCD once I start studying a subject. What follows, until I get to the recipes, are some of the discoveries I have made about grains in the last few years. If you don't have a similar geek bump on your DNA, you may want to skip this.

Besides feeling smug, I hope you are noticing a few other things changing. Four years ago, when I began to look for my own answers to why I couldn't regain my health, the first really big change for me was to eliminate grains. I know I am repeating myself, but modern grains have very little similarity to the grains from even fifty years ago. Dr. William Davis, author of 'Wheat Belly: Lose the Wheat, Lose the Weight, and Find Your Path Back to Health' is one of the best documented voices in the anti-grain movement. I recommend his book for a thorough assessment of the role of wheat in our collapsing national health. When he was diagnosed with Type Two Diabetes, he found little support was offered by the traditional medical community other than prescriptions. He began to look for answers, and by changing his diet, was able to overcome the diabetes.

Another excellent book is 'Grain Brain,' by Dr David Perlmutter. I have enjoyed two seminars with Dr. Perlmutter; he is a fine and entertaining speaker and tolerates questions well. His background is unique, as he began his medical career in neurology, and then earned a degree in nutrition. A rare combination! His father was also a neurologist, until he developed Alzheimer's. It was this that prompted David to study the correlation between neurological issues and diet, and from there to grains. A very readable and entertaining book, and available from my web site. www.Austin-Nutritional-therapy.com

Grains are problematic. They are very high on the glycemic index, meaning that they raise blood sugar more quickly than sugar. A baguette has an index of 95, while Coca Cola has an index of 63.[1] This means that a couple of slices of bread on a sandwich drive blood sugar higher and more quickly than a candy bar. Next time you are at a restaurant, look at the tables of other diners. It is rare that you see a meal in this country without a large portion of wheat.

Grains are mono-cropped. If you have ever driven across the Midwest, you have no doubt noticed the mile after mile of corn and wheat fields. 'America's Bread Basket' has brought forth an enormous amount of grain in the last fifty years. This has both degraded the mineral content of the soil, and led to terrible erosion in many areas. No minerals in the soil mean no minerals in the bread.

Science is finally conceding that cholesterol is not the enemy in cardiac disease. The 'Lipid Theory' put forth by Ancel Keys has been largely debunked, (available on my site, check out my book 'The Nutritarian Notebook' for Keys' story and his contribution to the great American cholesterol myth), but there is an element of cholesterol that is a reliable predictor of heart health: the increase of the dense, small molecules of LDL. This may be triggered by a starch in wheat, Amylopectin A. This is also the reason for the high glycemic rating as

26

this starch is the most rapidly absorbed.

Much has been written lately about 'carb addiction' which can be blamed on the gliadins in wheat. Studies have shown that this protein can have an opiate like effect on our brains. Gliadin is also the problematic element in Celiac disease, which often goes undiagnosed for years, wreaking havoc with digestive systems. Once thought to be rare, this autoimmune disease is being diagnosed more frequently, perhaps due to our development of grains containing much more starch than in the past.[2] Other genetic manipulations of grains, beginning in the 1970s, have altered the amino acid balance in grains, creating what is colloquially known as 'Frankengrains'. Our digestive systems, however, haven't been able to keep up that well. Wheat is added to many packaged foods, often under convoluted pseudonyms, to keep us eating 'just one more.'

Wheat has an estrogenic effect, increasing estrogen levels in men and women both, which can have consequences for reproductive cancers, such as breast, ovarian, uterine and prostate as well as lowered testosterone in men. The speedily absorbed starch is believed to be one of the main causes of belly fat. Insulin Resistance, aka Adrenal Fatigue, aka Metabolic Syndrome and our national obesity problems appear to have a very solid foundation in our wheat consumption. For an excellent and highly entertaining explanation of how this works, watch Tom Naughton's film: 'Fathead.' www.fathead-themovie.com.

Plants, being lousy warriors, and slow as well, developed other defenses, notably lectins. All seeds have some lectin, but grains and legumes are the seeds we consume in quantity. If you have ever eaten lettuce or perhaps basil after it has blossomed and gone to seed, it is very bitter. That is the flavor of lectin. Besides causing problems in our intestines, the lectin also makes it impossible to digest the seed. After all, the plant grew the seeds to propagate itself, not to feed us. (Lectins are also used as powerful insecticides.) If it can skate through our entire

27

system, it can still germinate. Most cultures have traditions of soaking, fermenting or sprouting seeds to eliminate at least some of the toxins, but these are methods used in times when we had little but grains between us and the wolf at the door. Sally Fallon Morel's book, 'Nourishing Traditions' has perhaps the best history and preparation methods for grains.

As stated in the very beginning of Perlmutter's book, grains are known to be inflammatory, and the whole point of this effort you are making is to *reduce* inflammation!

Leaky gut syndrome is being diagnosed more often with each passing year. The culprit appears to be agglutinin, found in the wheat germ, which can loosen the barriers in the small intestines, and leak into the bloodstream, causing havoc and the start of many autoimmune diseases.

If this is of interest, Sayer Ji of www.greenmedinfo.com has a lot more information on his site.

> 1 Harvard Health Publications, Harvard Medical School.
> 2 Dr. Joseph Murray, gastroenterologist, Mayo Clinic

End of Geek Alert…..

Enough already! Like most foods that are refined, there is a lot hidden beneath the benign face we see in advertisements. I feel sure that the opiate-like qualities of these foods have kept us from looking more closely at them, but now that you have been away from grains for almost a week, take some time to see if you feel any different. My experience was an immediate reduction in 'brain-fog.' My blood sugar began to stabilize soon after, and I found that my sense of being constantly hungry almost totally disappeared. Happily, my joint pain eased a lot, and while I had never felt that I was depressed, my happiness quotient shot up. I quickly lost my 'carb cravings' and began to crave fresh vegetables. If you know me at all, you know this was an enormous change. All this, I am reading from my journal of the first month I was away from the grains.

Four years later, I believe that I am healing still. There was a time when even a tiny amount of flour would trigger a reaction, and I understand now that there is something of a bell curve in healing. As I got away from eating grains, my sensitivity increased, as I quit creating all the compensating defenses for their toxicity. Then as my health improved, my tolerance got better. I have lost my taste for it, and seeing someone eating a sandwich on a slab of bread the size of a sofa cushion is a little queasy making, but I no longer have to skip a piece of birthday cake.

Back to the question of 'If I can't have a sandwich, or noodles or pizza, how is life worth living?' I've been there, and the first few weeks can be difficult. Not because I missed the grains so much as the darned inconvenience! I began to see how our entire diet is designed, not for health, but to make profits for the Foodopolies! Convenience is a luxury, and a little too costly in terms of my health to make it justifiable. And it isn't really an issue of convenience so much as habit. Pouring a bowl of cereal is no easier than pouring a smoothie.

Noodles I miss, especially Asian noodles. As grains go, rice is the most benign, issues of arsenic aside. Texturally, rice noodles, being free of gluten, don't have the same mouth feel as other pastas, and are better in Asian dishes. If you are dealing with blood sugar issues or trying to lose weight, this isn't a good option.

Spaghetti squash is another option, but I am not fond of the whole 'fake food' idea. By this I mean the idea that a non-grain 'bread' can be made that will taste like a French baguette. Squash is squash, and expecting it to taste like an al dente pasta is sure to disappoint. But a

29

nice baked casserole with a marinara sauce on squash with some lovely chopped basil is a fine dinner, with a salad, and when you start adding dairy into your life once more, some *pecorino Romano* is the perfect touch.

If you have a sauce recipe that fits into your current regime, think about using it on a vegetable. A vegetable peeler makes thin strips of zucchini, which can be boiled for a couple of minutes just to soften, then tossed with a little good olive oil, some garlic and black pepper. Marinara works well. Steamed cauliflower, chopped up and tossed with a sauce is lovely, and surprisingly good cooked *ala carbonara:*

Cavolfiore Carbonara

to serve 2

Small head of cauliflower

4 strips bacon

2 eggs, beaten

2 cloves garlic, chopped

1 Tablespoon olive oil

Handful chopped parsley

Steam the cauliflower and chop into florets. Put into serving bowl and cover to keep hot. In a skillet, over medium heat, cook the bacon until crisp, remove and crumble over the cauliflower. Reserve a Tablespoon of the rendered fat, and add the olive oil to the skillet. Put back on the heat and cook the garlic until golden. Add to the cauliflower and toss well, then add the eggs and toss until the cauliflower is evenly coated. If the eggs are not cooked as well as you like, place in a 350° oven for a few minutes. Top with parsley and serve. Of course, if you find that you tolerate dairy well, parmesan is wonderful on this.

Phase One, Day Six

Are we having fun yet? I always think of this way of eating as a challenge, kind of like the competitions on the Food Network. The fun of it is creating tasty meals within the restrictions. I'll bet it is getting easier isn't it?

Most of us are rocketing out of the house first thing in the morning, so the ease of the whey shakes often ends up making them breakfast. But if you began your detox on Monday, today is Saturday. Maybe it is a good time to break from the routine and have a more extravagant breakfast. Since you have been working hard all week, a relaxing meal, dawdling with the paper and planning how you are going to relax and play over the weekend can even be key to your success. Sure, it is a necessity, along with the massage you have planned for this afternoon...

Weekend breakfast in my family usually meant pancakes, waffles and such. But what is really better than steak and eggs? I have talked a little about sourcing clean, grass fed meats, which are getting easier to find. And yes, it is more expensive, but here is what I have found: whereas my husband and I in the past could devour a pound of steak each as a celebratory meal, if we get the much more nutritious grass fed meat, 4-6 ounces is quite a party. You are what you eat, and the commercial beef producers have no shame in feeding their animals cheaply, as well as feeding them food additives, hormones, and antibiotics to *make them fat.* Yes, you are what you eat, and everything the beef cattle in the feed lots are getting, you are getting.

While I have struggled over the decades with the ethical questions of eating meat, the truth is that we are consuming other's lives no matter what we eat. Grain for example. Simply plowing a field destroys lives, habitats and food sources for wildlife. Nests are destroyed, underground homes are ripped open. And as we continue monocropping grains, the biodiversity that had been a delicate balance

31

disappears. Row cropping, the technical word for growing most fruit and vegetable plants, is more intensive, but acre for acre, much more profitable and sustainable.

As to herding, there is a brilliant man who has done groundbreaking work in grassland ecosystems, especially in Zimbabwe. He has discovered a method for arresting desertification, and reversing it. Imagine a way to reverse global warming, feed people and make a profit. And yes, it involves herding. Google Alan Savory and watch a 15 minute talk on TED for a succinct explanation. Manure is the foundation of any farm, and we are not treasuring ours...

Steak and eggs then. A high density protein meal is a grand way to get the weekend going. But it can be a little heavy, so I like to make a base of roasted mushrooms. And when I bother with this, I make a lot and freeze it.

Roasted Mushrooms

2 pounds of mushrooms, whichever type you like, cleaned and sliced

Olive oil (perhaps with a little truffle oil...)

Chopped garlic to taste

Salt and pepper

Chopped parsley, thyme and/or marjoram (again, what you like)

Preheat your oven at 500°. Get out an ovenproof skillet, ideally cast iron. This is not the place for anything with a non-stick coating and plastic handle. You are, literally, going to be playing with fire. Put the skillet in the oven to heat up while you are preparing everything.

When the skillet has had at least fifteen minutes in the oven at full heat, toss in the mushrooms. Close the oven door and set the timer for 4 minutes. (I know, the temptation to add the oil is almost overwhelming, but believe me, they won't stick, and they will lose all their water, making them thirsty. When you add the seasoning and oil they will suck it up like little vacuums.) In four minutes, stir the mushrooms, keeping in mind that your oven is **500°**! Yes, that heavy duty pot holder is a Fine Idea. Set the timer again for four minutes; stir the seasonings into the oil in a bowl large enough to hold all of the 'shrooms. When the timer goes off, stir them again. You are looking for a fine, toasty caramelization. If the mushrooms were a little older they may be done- the fleshier mushrooms like criminis take a little longer, oyster mushrooms you might need to check after just a couple of minutes. Because of this, if I am using a variety of mushrooms, I may work in batches.

When they are the warm earth tones and gold that you like pull them out using the same heavy duty hot pad and dump them in the bowl. Move the still screaming hot skillet back into the oven, which you have turned off, so that no one can burn themselves. Toss the mushrooms, and if you like, this is a wonderful meal by itself. Add a little organic, pasture fed butter or cream when you aren't on the cleanse, and you have a nice Stroganoff. Add a little more dairy and you have cream of mushroom soup that Mr. Campbell would never recognize. And of course, if you have company, tossing a shot of brandy into the skillet as it comes from the oven is terrifically entertaining. Do tilt the skillet away from you, so that the brandy ignites on the side away from you.

As I mentioned, for a more leisurely meal, just pull a package of the already roasted mushrooms from the freezer on Friday night. I also like to salt and pepper and olive oil my steak the night before. Use more sea salt, like the Pink Himalayan or Real Salt than you think you need. As with the roasted chicken, there is a mechanical element going on here and it won't be too salty. If you are not a purist, some fresh thyme and/or rosemary, a little garlic or onion is always lovely.

33

If you are moving on to steak, take that out of the refrigerator as soon as you are in the kitchen. In half an hour it will be room temperature, which will ensure much more even cooking. If you have just cooked the mushrooms, you already have your grill ready! Get your hot pad and move the skillet to the hottest burner on your stove. Since you are going to have eggs as well, I recommend splitting a small ribeye or hanger steak with someone. If you don't have an appreciative live in person, offering breakfast on a Saturday morning, no strings attached, might be a step in that direction. When the skillet is again up to red hot (exhaust fan time) toss in the steaks. In 1 minute, flip them. In another minute, I think it is perfectly rare but for a more medium rare to medium, drop the heat or put them back in the still hot oven, but monitor the temperature with a thermometer. 135 ° is medium rare. It is also useful to learn how to tell doneness by touch. This also looks really cool. Hold out your hand, palm up. Touch the flesh at the base of your thumb. This is how raw steak feels. If you pull your index figure to touch the tip of your thumb, the same place feels like a medium rare steak. Your middle finger is a good medium, ring finger is medium well, and finally touching your pinkie to your thumb will give you the texture of well done. As will the sole of your shoe.

Before your steak is perfectly cooked, take it out of the pan and onto a plate, and cover. This is called 'resting' and will bring the meat's temperature up about 5 more degrees. It also allows the juices to redistribute in the meat. If you skip this part, the steak will dry out when you make the first cut and release the juices, which are bubbling away inside. Let it rest while you turn your attention to the eggs.

I like to sneak another serving of vegetables into scrambled eggs. Spinach is a natural, and you will be astounded by how much raw spinach cooks down. I use a cast iron *comal* which is like a skillet with no sides. It is probably the most used pan in my kitchen. Heat a bit of coconut oil or whatever you like and add some chopped garlic or onion. When it has just started to turn golden, add as much spinach as you can keep in the pan. Keep it moving with a pair of tongs and in seconds you will have a tiny little wad and some water as the spinach gives up its juice. Pour this off, but save it, if you are like me, to add to soup. At the very least, pour it over the dog's food. Drain in a strainer or on a paper towel. If you are using thawed frozen spinach, you will need to drain it too.

Add the spinach back to the pan, pour your scrambled eggs over, and stir gently over low to medium heat. Pull them off the stove before they are done and they will cook more as you plate them. A nice layer of mushrooms under the steak, eggs on the plate, and a bottle of Sriricha is a terrific and nutritionally dense way to get the weekend started. Plus you have already had at least two servings of vegetables.

Phase One, Day Seven

You are almost through the week. Wow. Has it been easier than you expected? Tougher? What are the hardest parts? Lots of things to journal about... The best part, that I have used continually, even after I finished the first thirty days, has been the big glass of water with lemon before anything else in the morning.

Journaling has been a part of my life since I was 14. Journaling about my health, my food, my exercise and my sleep habits, and comparing them to my regular journal has been revealing. For instance, if I want to sleep well, I have to get a minimum of 30 minutes of exercise that day. Swimming is best for me, but anything to get some blood flowing, and also, to move in a rhythm for a while works... Of course, I knew that in theory, but I think we 21st century humans really 'get it' better when we see something on a computer printout. Now I am using a check list similar to what you are filling out every night, which makes comparisons easier. This whole nutrition thing is infinitely complex, and I am still very much in learning mode. I love how the elimination aspects of the detox allow everyone to learn and tweak around exactly what they need. I don't know any other way to do it so precisely.

There are as many reasons to decide to do a detoxification program as there are people. And most people, like me, have several reasons. It has not been a real weight loss program for me, as the basic diet is almost identical to what I eat anyway. I found that the program was an end in itself, just for how happy and healthy it makes me feel. At the end of my first round, I was sorely tempted to keep going indefinitely. I decided to let my body recover for a few weeks before starting again. The constant influx of enzymes and other digestive aids and support for moving things out of my body is a lot of work for my whole system. I find that even knowing when I need to rest is still a steep learning curve for me!

A month later, I did another thirty days, and found the experience different. I still felt great by the middle of the first week, and comfortable with the regime, but the changes were more subtle. I was sleeping and eating well when I went in to it, so the immediacy was lost a little. It was comfortable and familiar. The third time, I started just after the holidays. While I did pretty well with the food and drink aspects, holidays are stressful, and body chemistry changes are stressful. A bad boss, traffic, and mustard gas all create similar chemicals in our bodies, which saturate every cell. I suppose I shouldn't have been surprised that the first week of the detox had a profound effect. My birthday is the end of January, so I timed it perfectly to be in great shape for the celebration!

This time, I also made some new changes. The regime stayed the same, but I tried to indulge myself more. It still feels a little like self-denial when I start and indulgences in other aspects of my life is a fine way to balance things. Of course, many of the 'indulgences' can carry over into some lovely habits. I set the table for meals, or eat on the deck. Mom's good silver is out and used daily. I bother with things like fresh flowers and music in the house. And I get much more conscientious about meditation. As long as I am in 'change mode' I want to take advantage.

I mentioned early on that it is a good idea to turn off your screens an hour before bed time. The light that our ancestors were used to is amber in the evening, which stimulates production of melatonin. Many people have used melatonin supplements to facilitate sleep. Done occasionally, for example when traveling, this can be benign (although be certain of your source). But if it is used for more than a few evenings in a row, it can actually suppress the body's production. After all, if there is plenty available, why bother to make more? Unfortunately the screens we so adore, like computers, tablets, e-books and such (and phones too) emit a bluish light, the color of dawn, which stimulates cortisol, aka the stress hormone, to wake us up. This goes a long way towards explaining the marathon television and video game sessions.

As long as you are turning off the screens and grabbing a book an hour before bed, consider a full media fast. Seriously. Think about one day a week when you don't use your phone, watch television or check your e-mail. At first this seems as difficult as giving up grains, but now that you are heading into the second week, that isn't as unthinkable, is it? And amazingly, Facebook will still be there the next day. Something to think about...

Another thing. It seems almost unpatriotic to eschew any freedom, but I have been giving far too much brain space and time and energy to petty decision making. Knowing that my breakfast shake, prepared in under a minute, plus my supplements are on the kitchen counter, ready to go, saves me about half an hour of decisions, cooking, cleanup and general bother, and I know that the whey shake will have me energized and clearheaded for the next few hours. Without caffeine! Life is simplifying....

Broccoli has a well-earned reputation as a powerhouse of nutrition. Here is an Italian preparation that is delicious, and no one will know your secret ingredient, which adds a ton of flavor and some wonderful Omega 3s. This will also serve two as an entrée or more as a side dish.

Broccoli con Acciughe

1/4 cup olive oil

1 Tablespoon capers

3 cups broccoli florets, washed and trimmed

1 tin excellent quality anchovies in olive oil

1 or more minced garlic cloves

Fresh black pepper

Juice of a lemon

Handful of Kalamata olives (optional)

Heat a heavy skillet over medium high heat. Add the oil, swirl to cover the bottom of the pan, and toss in the capers. They will snap and crackle and open up, then add the florets. Toss quickly, so they don't burn and once they begin to brown, add as many of the anchovies* and as much of the garlic as you like. Toss in the olives if you like. Keep stirring until the anchovies 'melt,' add the pepper, then plate and serve. Squeeze the lemon over the top. If you like add Parmesan. This with a salad is remarkably satisfying.

*Anchovies are largely known for messing up pizzas, but they are in fact, nutritional powerhouses, crammed with lovely fatty acids and Vitamin D. They are very low on the food chain, and as such, are one of the best and cleanest sources of seafood. Ortiz is the Dom Perignon, with a firm texture and mellow saltiness, but there are other good brands out there. Look for Mediterranean production and packaging in olive oil. These are your protein in the dish, so feel free to splurge a bit. And if you don't tell anyone they are in the broccoli, no one will know.

Phase Two, Day 8

Have you ever noticed in the old myths and fairy tales that the-magical objects are almost always from plants? Snow White's mother didn't give her a poisoned pork chop, Cinderella's coach wasn't made out of a chicken and Paris had a Golden Apple, not a barbecued rib. When Athena struck the ground with her staff, an olive tree sprouted, not a side of beef. The same is true in nutrition. Meat and all proteins supply a lot of re-building and repair elements, minerals, vitamins, but the real magic is in plants.

Centuries ago, in every culture, there was an herbal tradition. Before we could synthesize drugs from petroleum and such, we used an enormous pharmacopeia of plants. These traditions were handed down the generations and refined, and have given us the foundation of modern drugs. If you are using food-based supplements, and read the labels, you may be surprised by the plant names you recognize. Oregano oil, for example, has powerful anti-biotic, anti-fungal and anti-viral properties and has been used since very early times. Biotics Research uses it in a product called ADP, and Standard Process includes it in their Gut Flora Complex. While it works very much like pharmaceutical antibiotics, it has only rare side effects, (pizza breath) and does not damage the natural gut flora in the same way. Why then would we choose to use this rather than just get a prescription? That is an interesting question....

When grocery shopping, how do you choose your produce? First you look at it: say a stack of cantaloupe before you. When you spot one that appeals, you lift it, feeling for soft spots. Heavy for its size means riper, and then you probably smell it. If you are shopping at a higher end store, you may even be able to taste the goods. It is these old senses that let us know if food is good, and perhaps also, if it is the particular food we need. The information is available to us through every sense, every perception, if we can quiet ourselves enough to listen. . We are invested in reading as a source of knowledge, and we look for authorities to inform us, but we are also blessed with a solid intuition based on subtle sensory clues. Without a cell phone or a schedule, I would suggest these clues might be much easier to read. You have an exquisitely refined, phenomenally sensitive piece of equipment attached directly to the front of your face. Use it!

Centuries ago, in both the Old and the New Worlds, most of the healers were women. While men, as Shamans, carried on the spiritual and religious aspects of a culture, women, perhaps because they often stayed closer to the hearth, did the day to day care of the sick, the elderly, the injured and the infants. From Bronze Age and earlier burials, we know that men were frequently buried with spears and other weapons suitable for war and hunting large animals. Women on the other hand, had digging sticks, snares and slings in their graves. It is not so surprising then, that medicine bags, and ancient collections of herbs were most frequently found buried with the older women of a tribe. These women were the midwives and herbalists and were highly valued for their wisdom.

Then with the rise of the university system, the illiterate women who were often barred from education lost favor as doctors, educated and powerful, often from wealthy families, began to take over the practice of medicine. The widespread condemnation of the Old Wisdom, aka witchcraft by the church, drove the surviving practitioners underground, and a lot of the knowledge was lost.

In India, Ayurvedic Medicine has been practiced for centuries. It was first recorded in the Veda, the world's earliest known literature, after centuries of being passed on through the oral tradition from teacher to student, and spread very early to China and beyond. We have only begun to accept the precepts of Ayurveda in Western Medicine, and delve into a richness of traditions very different from our ideas of medical practice.

Given the centuries of knowledge, why has medicine as we understand it in the West become almost entirely identified with the alleviation of symptoms with pharmaceuticals? I would suggest that it is a love affair that began early in the twentieth century with the Miracle Drug, penicillin, and continued with the miracle of Salk's polio vaccine. What could have empowered the MDeities more than suddenly being able to literally heal people overnight, as well as create an immunity and eliminate scourges like smallpox?

It has not been the judicious use of antibiotics that has brought about the new antibiotic resistant bugs, but rather their usage with factory raised meat such as chickens, pigs and beef. In the 80's it was discovered that animals fed a steady diet of antibiotics would gain weight. (And we can certainly guess that it has a similar effect on humans.) It also allowed the animals to be raised in horrific conditions, on the assumption that they could not get sick. We consume the meat, and also the antibiotics. Perhaps the single best thing you can do for your health is to establish a relationship with the people where you buy your proteins. Sustainably and humanely raised animals may be more expensive, but for change to happen it is crucial that the smaller, more intensively caring farmers have our support. And again, you will find that meat that is full of nutrients from animals that were cared for is more satisfying than a much larger serving of factory raised meat. And it also is light years more delicious.

The upshot perhaps being this: It may be a good thing to look at alternatives for your health care with respect. Not everyone works the same way. Like corporate food, corporate medicine may not make my health and well-being as much of a priority as the bottom line. This year, 2014, will be the first year that Integrative Medicine will be licensed as a specialty in Texas. This is a milestone, because it reverses the traditional western medicine view that it can provide all the answers regarding health care.   It is time to lose the idea that health consists of simply not being sick.

Fresh Herb Salad

1 Bunch of Parsley, Chopped

12 Large Fresh Basil Leaves, Torn into small bits

Juice of ½ Lemon

Lemon Zest

3 Large Sprigs of Thyme

1 Large Tomato, diced

1 Large Green Onion, Chopped

½ Cup Olive Oil or MCT Oil*

Salt and Pepper to Taste

This is so much more than a salad; it's a prescription. Once all of the fresh herbs and veggies are chopped, simply stir everything together and keep covered in the fridge. Herbs have a wonderful way of helping move toxins out of the body, so use this salad as freely as you choose. It can be a topping for broiled fish or chicken, an addition to romaine as a full salad, or in a lettuce wrap as a chimichurri. It can be eaten by itself, or you can substitute lime and cilantro for lemon and parsley. Feel free to play around with the ingredients as you choose! If there are specific herbs you like, try them out in different combinations in this salad. The softer herbs like basil, cilantro and parsley are full of chlorophyll which supports detoxification, so use this salad with abandon.

*MCT or Medium Chain Triglyceride is the very best part of coconut oil. Elaine and I both love it in coffee. It is very bland, so a good oil for salad dressing or mayonnaise. Does NOT do well when heated so it is not recommended for cooking. Since it is tasteless, it is remarkable for absorbing flavors like fresh herbs and expanding them, rather than interfering with them.

Phase Two, Day Nine

With the huge kerfuffle over Obama Care, (and personally, I really don't think the 2014 winter storms were caused by Obama Care) much of our 'Health Care System' has been scrutinized. Make no mistake, it is not a health care system, it is a sick care system. And it isn't even very good at that, according to the standards of most industrialized countries. As a 'for profit' system, it focuses, much more on keeping the pharmaceutical companies wealthy than on keeping the general population healthy. But I also feel the paradigm that we have been sold; that a symptom is not a signal of an underlying problem, but rather an opportunity for medication, is the most destructive element.

Don't get me wrong! Modern western medicine has a great deal to recommend it, particularly in the areas of trauma care. Without modern medicine I would likely have died at 28 and then again in my thirties. My husband, Don, had a massive heart attack on October 22, 2014, was dead for around 12 minutes, had a triple bypass, and was walking a mile a day within a month. I am grateful. Without CPR, a defibrillator, a talented surgeon and the fact that when Don fell from the Lucky Tree he hit every branch on the way down, he would not be here. And the elimination of smallpox and polio, the enormous gift of antibiotics, (at least until we started overusing them) and anesthesia are all huge advances. It is the idea that by taking a pill, we can resolve a problem without being inconvenienced that I find disturbing.

There are many other health care disciplines that work to achieve optimal health, all less convenient than taking a pill. I find that when someone wants to engage a nutritional therapist they usually have a specific symptom that they want to address. I blame the medical model that we have been taught for this mindset. While herbal and nutritional remedies have fewer side effects than most pharmaceuticals, the basis of nutritional therapy is to use food and sometimes supplements to

45

build health, which addresses the underlying problems, and the symptoms go away.

Here's an example: A client starts out with me, and in the beginning paperwork, I ask about symptoms. This woman has insomnia. She wants me to recommend a brand of melatonin. Looking at her information, I feel certain that her problem is a volatile blood sugar level. She has been working into the night, then watches television or works at her computer when she gets home, disrupting her sleep cycle. She often works weekends and doesn't make time for rest, exercise, or relaxation. Most of her meals are eaten in her car. My suggestions would involve a lot of changes, and not easy ones. Or she could take an over the counter 'sleep aid' with a long list of side effects. Hmmmm. Which way do you think that one is going to go?

Of course we see this over and over with friends and family who have a life threatening illness scare. I know now that prior to my devastating accident, I had a lot of 'wake-up; calls; The Fall was a last ditch effort by my body to MAKE me slow down, sip the coffee, smell the roses...

I have taken a couple of classes from Dr. Court Vreeland, who runs a lovely clinic in New England, www.vreelandclinic.com, where he specializes in neurological disorders. I was fascinated, and impressed with his sweeping knowledge and understanding of underlying causes that can precipitate many neurological problems, from depression to MS to dementia and Parkinsons. His theory is that we all have a 'tipping point'. As the stress builds, as it is with my insomniac client from the last paragraph, we scramble to cope with increasing problems, until we are overwhelmed and go into a more serious disease process. Our individual tipping point. There may be a genetic element, as there seems to be with some cancers, but environmental and lifestyle choices appear to be a much greater influence. For example, a heavy smoker, coming from a family that carries a lot of dementia, will probably develop pulmonary problems first. His tipping point would be

46

influenced primarily by how much he smoked. We are seeing this now with the 'obesity epidemic.' The lack of healthy, fresh, nutritionally dense food and the propagandizing of fast food, breakfast cereals, and other food like substances are herding us into making a lot of bad choices at mealtime, resulting in obesity and diabetes and a host of other issues.

Picture a seesaw. You are sitting on one end, and your bad choices are piling up on the other. As time passes, you are lifted higher and higher. When the other end of the seesaw touches the ground, you are at your tipping point. This is when most people ask for help. But if you can lighten up the other end of the seesaw, even a little, you may be able to pull back from a serious disease. The job of any health care provider is to help you do exactly that.

And it isn't easy. We are pushed from all sides to consume. Most of the marketing is for products that few people would ever buy if they knew the truth about them. We put an inordinate amount of faith in regulating agencies that are often controlled, if not outright owned by the corporations making the profits. This isn't new; corruption and greed probably started about the time we began walking upright. 'The Jungle' an expose of slaughterhouses in Chicago was written in 1906. The information is out there, but it is buried under an avalanche of KFC boxes.

Change is hard for everyone, especially when the change involves giving up comfort. David Kessler's book, 'The End of Overeating in America' discusses the extremes of the food industry, developing more and more addictive products. The addition of hydrogenated vegetable fats, refined sugars, chemicals and salt that are diabolically layered for maximum effect is especially scary. He discusses something called 'the bliss point,' the Holy Grail of food engineers. This is the balance of ingredients that creates cravings and morphine like addictions.

We have evolved to seek out the maximum calories and nutrients from foods that require the least work. All animals incorporate this programming or they wouldn't survive. We are in essence lazy and hungry. Suddenly we are surrounded by intensely caloric and accessible food with very little effort at all on our part. And there is aggressive competition on the part of the producers to sell us their particular product. By engineering the food like substances to make them more and more addictive, the producers are also raising the bar for intensity. The detox you are doing right now is deprogramming a lot of what the Standard American Diet has uploaded to you. It is not unlike a steady diet of rap music at maximum volume suddenly being turned off. It may take a few hours, but eventually you will be able to hear birdsong again.

Salsa (Persimmon/Peach)

1 lb Tomatoes, diced

1 Medium Bell Pepper, seeded and finely diced

2 Jalapenos, seeded and finely diced

1 Medium Onion, finely diced

1 1/2 lbs Peaches, diced, or Fresh Persimmons

1/2 Bunch of Cilantro, chopped

5 Tbsp lime juice

1 1/2 tsp salt, or to taste

We are so lucky to live in the South. We have peaches and persimmons! Persimmons add a richness to the salsa that makes it much heartier, and slightly more sweet. Feel free to add more lime juice to complement the level of the sweetness of any fruit you use.

Phase Two, Day 10

With my husband Don's heart attack this year, I have done a lot more reading about cardiac health. He was so very lucky, being with friends, one of whom was able to do CPR (Thanks Johnathan!). He was shouting distance from a fire station, and within a couple of miles of Austin's Heart Hospital. We had returned from a bicycling trip to West Texas just a couple of hours earlier, where he had spent hours, at altitude, biking outside of range for cell phones. He was wearing a helmet, so no concussion when he hit the pavement. And he was in terrific shape. But he still had a heart attack.

The idea that a good diet, whatever that is, or an extreme exercise regime, or meditation or anything else can make you 'bulletproof' is a dangerous one. Everyone has a different equilibrium and it is going to inexorably shift throughout our lives. Worshiping at the altar of exercise, without quality rest and fuel is the current fashion, and we are paying for it. Over the twenty plus years that I spent working for the YMCA here in Austin, I saw many athletes dedicate themselves to aerobic fitness at the cost of their joints. Hearts and lungs don't maintain those exquisite aerobic levels very long at all when you are nursing a knee surgery, as I found first hand.

One third of the way through this endeavor, what have you learned? If you sleep better, are you less likely to eat badly? If you get a 20 minute nap in the afternoon, or meditate, does your energy production increase or decrease? If you walk at lunch time, because you packed a lunch and only took a few minutes to eat, how does the rest of the day go? Now, while you are in the midst of this accelerated learning about yourself and what you need to optimize your existence, what would you like to remind yourself of six months from now?

Interesting work on cardiac health from the University of Connecticut found that people who deliberately set out to be grateful and especially to express gratitude to others improved their physical and emotional health, and if they were at risk for heart disease, lowered that risk. It is also one of the best ways to manage stress. The old Bing Crosby song from the film 'White Christmas' was before its time.

"If you are worried and you can't sleep

Count your blessings instead of sheep.

You'll fall asleep, counting your blessings..."

Technology gives us some great advantages in this area. Cell phone alarms can be set to remind us of gratitude, and can jolt us out of negative and stressful thought patterns. Calendars can be handy for making notes, and thinking of a few things to be grateful for first thing in the morning can set a much gentler and less arduous tone for the day than the usual unattainable to-do list. While this may seem a little facile or superficial, resent studies in Cognitive Therapy show that the results can be profound.

Over my many years, I have known a number of dyed in the wool pessimists and lived with more than one. In my mind, it comes down to a control issue. I say the end of the world is next Tuesday at noon, and if I am wrong, everyone is happy and forgets, whereas if I am right, I am brilliant. Given the terrible toll of looking for the darkest side of everything, it is an expensive game and I suspect one misses a lot of rainbows and sunsets, not to mention mundane things that are transformed when one is grateful. Life transforming indeed.

Hence the questions in your evening paperwork regarding gratitude. When you are eating better, you are fitter emotionally, and when you are in a new mode of living, even temporarily, it is a grand time to move closer to the life would enjoy the most, by well, enjoying the life you have more!

I mentioned journaling a few chapters back, and a 'Gratitude Journal' is a fine practice to start. Joan Buchman, who suffers from fibromyalgia, an autoimmune disease that has been linked to grain consumption has written extensively about her journaling activities and the subsequent improvements in her health. www.cfidsselfhelp.org/library/the-healing-power-gratitude It is all about equilibrium. If it is a blizzard outside, instead of beating yourself up about not being able to get out for your usual run, try making a list of the ten things you are grateful for today. Take pictures on your camera. In looking for things to enjoy, you may be doing your heart more good than if you had gotten that run.

Hummus
1 Can (12oz) Organic Chick Peas

2 tbsp. Organic Tahini

4 Cloves Raw Garlic

Juice of 1 Lemon

¼ Cup Water

½ Cup Olive Oil

Salt to Taste

Rinse the chickpeas well under cool water. Place everything together in your food processor, or blender. Blend/Grind until smooth, about 3 to 5 minutes depending on the power of your machine and your preferred texture.   Open the top and taste it. Add what you think it needs. Blend again to mix and serve! This is also a condiment. Feel free to add this to salads, dip carrots in it for lunch, or use it instead of mayo in a lettuce wrap. You'll get the drift here once you taste it.

Phase Two, Day 11

With two of four meals taken care of, and your supplements neatly packed, things are getting easier. You are closing on the halfway mark, you have acquired some new cooking skills, delicious recipes are sparking your creativity, and you are feeling pretty good about things. Now you are going to cheat. And that isn't a failure or an excuse to quit. It is your body wanting to revisit foods that have worked for you in the past as comfort, or entertainment or that have just become habits.

Like sustainable agriculture, your food choices need to be sustainable. If you choose to only do the supplements and shakes and not change how you eat at all, you will still get some benefit from this detox. At the other end, if you follow orders like your life depends on it, you will get more benefits, of course, but you will also be shirking responsibility for your choices. Sustainability and reality are somewhere on that spectrum. I often, around this point in a client's detox, get a phone call asking for permission to do something that isn't on the protocol. The good news is: if you haven't cheated until now, a few bites of something *verboten* may not feel so good, and may not taste so good either. For the sake of staying in control, schedule something today or tomorrow. Keep it small, and pay close attention to how you react. A cookie maybe or a glass of iced tea sounds good. Does the cookie taste different from what you expected? Do you suddenly want another even more than you wanted the first? Does the caffeine hit you harder than it used to? All good information, and be sure to make a note on the questionnaire you fill out each evening.

Our culture places a lot of moral burden on how and what we eat. How often have you heard someone say, or said yourself: 'I can't have dessert; I am trying to be good.'? If guilt tripping yourself helps you make good choices, more power to you, but I find guilting myself to be very stressful. Make the food good or bad, or even better, make it food

52

and non-food. Instead of a phrase like: 'I am so bad, I ate the whole pint of Ben and Jerry's' you can go for the rigid: 'Ice cream is not something I eat. 'That works for me with things like my beloved Diet Coke. For something like ice cream, I use a different rationale: 'Ice cream is a celebration food, and today what I need is excellent fuel. Then when I am with others, and celebrating, ice cream will be appropriate.' I can save the foods that offer less than great nutrition for special occasions. And we all know that scarcity makes anything more valuable. Ice cream every night can actually get a little boring, but anticipating pumpkin pie with whipping cream through the entire month of November makes the pie Spectacular!

Almost everyone I have worked with through this detox protocol starts out with something non-negotiable. Often it is coffee (or Diet Coke) or a glass of wine to end the work day. What I have found is this: give yourself permission to have whatever you want that you feel you simply can't avoid for 30 days. Set limits. For example, instead of a bottle of wine at night, try having just a glass. Instead of a pot of coffee, perhaps two cups will do? If a sandwich for lunch is the only conceivable possibility, take off one slice of bread. This is surprisingly empowering. We have a tradition in our culture of helplessness, as though the Devil made you do it. Start a different tradition of being responsible and in charge of your choices. And each time you reach for whatever you have decided is necessary for your happiness, revisit it: 'Yesterday, I really needed my 3 p.m. candy bar from the vending machine, and the day before that and the day before that. Today, not so much. Maybe what I need is getting out of my chair and walking to the vending machine, and today I think I will take my walk outside instead.' Seriously empowering stuff, and it also draws your attention to what you actually need and away from habits that may not be serving you well. If, once you have gone through the entire month, and you find that even after close consideration, that Snickers bar seemed necessary every afternoon, let go of the guilt and stressing about it. There are worse things, certainly.

Here's how that works. As I mentioned, Diet Coke was my serious Jones. I still get one about every 6 months, and it gets increasingly less interesting. But on a hot day, I am driving home, and it starts to sound really good. I didn't bother to bring a meal with me, because I had expected to be back home in an hour, and now I am starving. And Sonic has half priced drinks in the afternoon. And there is one just down the street, that I am going right past. But I shouldn't have one! Why am I so weak? I know that the Nutrasweet turns to horrible things in my brain, and messes with my pancreas, but just one won't hurt, will it? Hell, I used to be a six pack a day girl and I haven't had one in a month….

See what is going on here? I am guilting myself into an anxiety attack. Just as the 12 step programs remind us, we are at our most vulnerable when we are at HALT: Hungry, Anxious/Angry, Lonely and Tired. In Texas in the summer, I would add Hot and Thirsty. I am talking myself into all of these things, so when I swerve through three lanes of traffic and into the Sonic lot, I am somewhere around HALT Cubed. I order my thrifty half priced drink, and since 'I am being bad' I add fries on also. I take the first gulp, and immediately feel the profound relief. Here's what happened: I have amped myself up so that the rush from the crap I am ingesting gives me a much more powerful pleasure rush than it would if I was at a party, for example, and to avoid the frozen margarita machine, I poured a half glass of Diet Coke and carried it around. What a terrific way to reinforce my addiction!

Once you grasp this scam, you will recognize it in a lot of advertising, as well as the behaviors of folks around you. If you make a happy and conscious decision to have a 'treat,' it is going to be much better for you if you congratulate yourself on a wise decision, decide exactly what it is you want, put yourself in a situation of maximum enjoyment, and savor that ice cream or Diet Coke or martini. Then walk away.

Broiled Fish w/ Chimichurri or Salsa

4 Filets of High Quality White Fish – Grouper, Snapper, Tilapia*

2 Tbsp. Coconut Oil

Salt and Pepper to taste

Salsa or Chimichurri to top

Toss the fish in the oil, add the salt and pepper, and arrange the fish on a heat proof pan at least a ¼ inch apart. Broil the fish about 3 inches from the heat source; probably the second highest rack in your oven. A general rule of thumb for broiling times is as follows: Allow 2 minutes per side for each 1/2-inch of fish thickness. The reason for high quality fish here is profound. So few ingredients allow you to enjoy the flavor of the seafood. Top the fish with the salsa or chimichurri to taste. You can even put the fish in a lettuce wrap with herb salad for fish tacos.

*One of the best things you can do for your health is to know where and how your protein is raised. Fish are often farmed, both here and overseas, and fed massive amounts of antibiotics, just as cattle are in feed lots, to compensate for the crowded conditions. Wild caught is but your fishmonger should also have the information. In 2002, COOL, aka Country of Origin Law, was passed in the United States, and every catch must be labeled. Avoid Chinese and Vietnamese sources in particular. Not only are they raised in terrible conditions, but they are also devastating the coastal environment in SE Asia. Like pasture raised farm animals, you will pay somewhat more, but nutritionally, wild caught is a bargain. Check www.montereybayaquarium.com to download their frequently updated and downloadable Seafood Watch.

Phase Two, Day 12

If you read the introduction to this book, you already know that this thirty day detox program is not a weight loss program. What you are in the middle of now is an attempt to rev up your body's ability to flush toxins out. Of course, those toxins weigh something, so it is likely that you will end up with a smaller number on the scale. There is also lots of evidence that it is so difficult to lose weight, especially if you are older, and/or a woman, because retaining fat helps disperse toxins, that we are wise enough not to want to dump back into our more bio-active bloodstream.

In my decades of struggling with my weight, I have tried just about every 'diet,' from vegetarian (gained weight) to Atkins (lost weight, then gained back more) to 'The Last Chance Diet' in the 70's which was similar to Atkins, but had a drink of predigested liquid protein as well. The same result as Atkins. Any of these diets, as well as Jenny Craig, Weight Watcher's (gained, gained) work well for some people, at least temporarily. In the long run, I believe that I carry about five extra pounds for every calorie restricted 'diet' I have tried. If you have watched the reality shows about weight loss, you have seen a graphic example of the shame our country has attached to overweight. The cultural belief system is simply: anyone who is overweight eats too much and moves too little because they have a weak character. If only it was that simple.

I have close to fifty years of experience with weight loss, and despite a daily effort, I am still wearing the same size I did thirty years ago. There have been episodes when I was a couple of sizes smaller, as well as the two years in a wheelchair weight gain that took me up two sizes. With all of that experience, this is how I believe it works: We survived into the mid-twentieth century by devoting most of our time and energy to

56

getting enough to eat. Our brains are formed with this compulsion, and for millennia, starvation and the proximity of famine was our main stressor. With the mass production of grains, with refrigeration and other preservation methods, and with breeding of plants to produce more, many of us have the strange privilege of food being overly available. Driving from San Antonio to Austin recently, about 100 miles, I was only out of sight of a sign advertising food or a place to buy food for a very few minutes. Imagine how active my old lizard brain was, responding to all of this stimulation!

Fearing starvation was how my ancestor's brains may have interpreted all stress. All of us have descended from a long line of famine survivors. What I believe happens in 2014 is a hyper awareness of the availability of food, plus a great deal more anxiety and pressure. My brain is then going to tell my endocrine system to slow down doing everything unnecessary and hang on to my fat, especially that good, accessible belly fat, to guard against the impending famine. Think about it. We now know that carbohydrates, delicious, and often occurring in tandem with some pretty nice nutrition, tend to put fat on our bellies. I have never heard of anyone with a 'beer thigh.' Until very recently, though, we only had access to carbohydrates in large quantities in the late summer and early fall, when we harvested fruit and grains. Beyond that carbs were from an occasional tuber, or the lovely happenstance of a honey cache. And what are we preparing for in the fall? Winter of course, when game is scrawny when it is available at all, and we rely on what food we have been able to preserve and store, including those carbs that we stored as belly fat. That impulse to nap after a big meal isn't just the tryptophan in the turkey or the boring football game. If I was going to make it through the winter 10,000 years ago, I needed to hang on to every calorie I could.

And our hardware hasn't changed much at all in that time. When we went from hunter-gatherers to farming, fossil evidence indicates that we lost a few inches in stature and some brain size. I guess tracking the wily hairy mastodon might have needed a little more strength and brain activity than plowing. But everything else still works pretty much the same. Our endocrine system gets excited by the prospect of a meal, and also helps us hang on to all of that lovely, life preserving fat. As a friend of mine said: 'Elaine, if it was 2000 years ago, you would be the grandmother rocking the babies by the fire, because all of the skinny grandmothers would be dead of starvation.' Perhaps we crones who can survive on small amounts of food, and in fact thrive, evolved with that ability to allow the young, strong people in the tribe to go out and hunt and gather, while we became the hearth watchers.

How does this translate today? It is difficult, when we are bombarded by images (photoshopped) of bizarrely slender people consuming all manner of food and drugs, with enormous smiles, to not succumb to the idea that we can torture our bodies into that fantasy. The predominant medical model is that we need to interfere and master our bodies in order to be healthy. My experience indicates that precisely the opposite is true. Our bodies know what they are doing, or they wouldn't have survived this long. (I dislike separating minds from bodies, but it is convenient to use 'mind' to mean the cognitive, logical overthinking part, and body to mean the intuitive, hormonal and perhaps wiser part.) If the myriad of stressors we are absorbing in the 21st century is interpreted as impending famine, our absolutely brilliant endocrine system is going to help us get as fat as possible.

What to do? Relaxing and managing your stress would seem paramount. Beyond that, trying to establish a dialogue between that gargantuan overthinking mind and the voice from within that really wants to be healthy is crucial. Our need for busy-ness or at least the appearance of busy-ness squelches that voice telling us we are tired, even exhausted. Sitting in a desk chair for hours on end is only doable if that little voice is ignored. And learning to hear what our bodies are actually hungry for takes focus. The blood sugar fluctuations that we give ourselves with the relatively new influx of refined carbohydrates

58

are what we interpret as hunger- low blood sugar. But if we normalize our food intake by eliminating the refined foods, the voice becomes much clearer. What is often called a low carbohydrate diet is in fact a normal carbohydrate diet.

As to the hyper stimulation of food advertising, it is actually pretty simple. We have learned very recently that Taco Bell, Nabisco and such sell food. It is a simple thing to unlearn this. They do not sell food, they sell foodish substances. This effectively negates food advertising. It is simply not food. I don't smoke, so a cigarette is irrelevant to me. In the same way, I don't eat fast food, and the glittering drive-thrus are not relevant either. Not Real Food. Hence this book, because if you want to eat real food, eventually it will dawn on you that you have to learn to cook. There are plenty of businesses out there who will be happy to take your money and damage your health, but it is not such a difficult thing to take back the control.

We believe that slenderness means health. Certainly it is better to not carry excessive weight, but at what cost? Denying your body the nutrition it needs, which is the foundation of the American Diet Industry, will ultimately make your body more desperate to gain weight. Perhaps it is time to relax, rest, exercise in a way that can be sustained, and make choices to prioritize health over weight. We all like to believe that we are unique, and by giving our bodies everything we can to make it happy and healthy, I believe we will evolve into the unique body we were born with.

Fritatta

6 eggs, beaten

1 -ounce Parmigiano-Reggiano, grated (optional)

1/2 teaspoon black pepper

Pinch salt

1 teaspoon coconut oil

1/2 cup boiled asparagus, chopped into ¼ lengths

1 tablespoon chopped parsley

Turn your oven's broiler to high, and set the rack about three inches from the heat source. Beat eggs, Parm, parsley, salt and pepper together. Boil the asparagus for 3 minutes, drain, and sauté in the coconut oil over medium heat until tender. Pour in egg mixture, and cook for 4 minutes or so. Make sure to use a rubber spatula to lift the egg gently as it cooks. This will allow the cooked egg underneath to fluff, and the raw egg to run down to the bottom of the pan. Place pan under your oven's broiler until eggs are puffy and cooked to your liking, about 2 to 4 minutes.

The glory of the frittata is that you can recycle any leftovers into the pan before the eggs. The combinations are endless, and you can use bits of leftovers to avoid wasting food! Don't be shy to use crazy ingredients, but make sure the leftovers are heated all the way through before you add the eggs. You should try this dish cold, as well. One can never underestimate the value of a grab and go breakfast from the fridge.

You're nearly through the second week, and now have a stack of questionnaires finished. What are you noticing? Is your sleep better? How about dreaming? How has your emotional status changed? If you are in general feeling happier, this could indicate that you have removed a food that was in fact stressing your system. If you have felt more anxiety during this process, it could be that food as a comfort was more important to you than you realized, and now is a fine time to explore other ways to nurture yourself. The coffee was something that I sorely missed the first time around, but I discovered that making the coffee, the ritual involved was a lot of what I loved. Grinding the beans, the smell, the comforting gurgle of the brewing, were all part of my morning routine. As soon as I went back to making a pot for my husband, and having my lemon water instead, missing the actual cup of java almost disappeared. You have a lot of information in your hands with the questionnaires and a lot of time, resources and motivation to make some choices to enhance your health long term. Take a look and see what has been changing for you. What is working, what can you tweak? The questionnaire is available from my site, www.austin-nutritional-therapy.com as a download that you can edit to better suit you. Consider it a rudimentary template.

Previously, I talked about relaxing and letting your body settle into its own ideal. I can't emphasize enough how valuable that idea is. We are bombarded by so many images of what a perfect, or even a 'good' body is, relentlessly, from every side. This does not actual serve us, but it DOES keep us dissatisfied with how we look and thus vulnerable to anyone with a new fashion, deodorant, or God help us, 'diet.' Does it strike you as odd that we all know that we are unique, that we flock to 'experts' who can tell us if we are a 'summer' or a 'spring' hoping that we can do the magical incantation with color that will make us uniquely beautiful, but when we see an ad for the new diet supplement, we

61

assume that it works well for everyone.

This program, I came to realize about halfway through the first time, is about integrity. It is the antithesis of taking the easy way, and assuming that what works for you will work for me. There are of course, some things that are universal. I doubt that processed and manufactured foods will ever be better for anyone than food from healthy, clean and well raised plants and animals. Beyond that very basic foundation, though, we are all so beautifully idiosyncratic! And this is such a powerful tool to really let those differences come to light! By eliminating many daily stresses and setting aside this month from the 'rest of your life' to prioritize health, you can discover what makes you, specifically, happy and healthy. And despite the urgings of practically everyone who has something they would like to sell you, you are the only one who can make that decision.

Living in a time when we have access to an endless stream of stuff, it is tempting to just buy the next cheap thing, try it and discard it if it doesn't work. This is what keeps the economy moving after all. It is as though we no longer have value as a voting citizen, but rather we have become useful only as consumers. Even if you are in the lucky position of not feeling the impact of this economic downturn, wouldn't you rather be saving money and time and energy rather than wasting it? And here we are back to integrity. What suits you? What are they trying to sell you? How will it fit into and enhance your life? Acquiring self-knowledge is the key to this wisdom, and you are in the belly of that beast. Keep up the questionnaires; they will become more and more valuable. And trust your innate wisdom.

In the west, we like to see things in opposites: black and white, good and evil. We worship concrete, Scientific Methodist style knowledge, and often ignore the more abstract and slippery wisdom of intuition. But in separating these two, we deny that they are in fact the same. Before a scientist can run an experiment, the intuition is necessary for how it will proceed. To learn a new fact or establish a theory, one must have direction. This is why double blinds and such are important in science. It is almost impossible to not read results in a way to support the desired findings.

When I started work on this project, I took copious notes on research, which I dearly love. But as I progressed, and pulled up scholarly papers from the Internet to support my experience, I also started to pull up similarly supported research that proved the opposite. This is a marketing executive's dream, because one day, the new big breakthrough can be sold aggressively while The Next Big Thing is readied in the wings, and if you can keep the stream moving, with lots of smoke and mirrors and sparkly things, very few people will notice that most of the Next Big Things are useless to almost everyone. Pick any health subject and Google it. I have yet to find a subject that doesn't appear to have concrete scientific evidence on both sides.

Ultimately, did it feel right to you? Determining that it made you feel good and calm and happy is a solid basis to support a decision that you make for yourself. Another good thing is to look at who funded the study if you want that sort of substantiation. Very little in the way of research is funded independently, and this has an enormous effect on the 'results.' Trying to find a study done in the United States on Genetically Modified Organisms that isn't funded somewhere down the line by Monsanto is quite a challenge, and how could it be otherwise, when they have the financial ability to support the research? The glut of information we are exposed to has to rely on sensationalism to get our attention, and often exploits a small piece of a study to get those headlines. But if it is something that will impact your health, I believe it is important to both read the research and listen to your intuition as well. Your gut feelings are a wonderful source of information. And seriously, did anyone ever prefer the taste of margarine to butter? Just because something is unpleasant doesn't mean it is good for you, and in fact, I would suggest that the opposite is true. Decisions based on

63

pleasure have always worked better for me.

Roasted Root Vegetables

4 large Carrots

4 large Parsnips

2 large Beets

2 large Onions

1 large sweet potato

1 large Turnip

2 tbsp. Olive Oil

1 tsp. Fresh Rosemary

½ Cup Bone Broth

Salt to taste

Preheat oven to 400 degrees. Peel all veggies and cut into ¼ inch squares. Don't worry if they're not perfect... We'll call it rustic. Toss the veggies in the salt and olive oil with the rosemary and place in a cast iron skillet. Bake for 30 minutes, stirring every ten to avoid sticking. Once roasted, add bone broth and cover. Allow to bake for another 30 minutes and you're done! Rich and delicious, this can be pureed with stock to make a root veg soup.

Phase Two, Chapter Fourteen

Stress is a good thing; without external stimulation, we don't grow and change. But often, it is too much of a good thing. Since you are spending much of this month eliminating food stresses, now is a good time to look at what else is making you crazy. Our world is hyper stimulating. As seemingly enjoyable as that is, it is also exhausting.

Meditation is an option. Since most of the things that give us a stress response are challenges from the environment or other people, taking a few minutes a day to settle in a quiet spot and cut out as much stimulation as possible is a necessity. There are as many ways to meditate as there are people. The simplest method for a beginner is just watching your breath. Sit comfortably, relax and watch your breath. In. Out. If you count ten breaths and get fidgety, then you can decide to be done for that session. If a mantra seems like a good idea, choose one. The word doesn't matter, according to 1975's 'Relaxation Response' by Herbert Benson. Over the forty plus years that I have meditated, I have changed mine more than once. While any word works, you are entraining your brain to relax in response to a particular word. I spend about twenty minutes once or twice a day meditating, and use the word 'relax' on the inhale and 'release' on the exhale. I have found this invaluable. When I encounter a need for serenity, a few exhales can help me release whatever is driving me nuts.

About five years ago, when I started trying to turn my brain into something useful rather than the puddle of polenta it had become, I came across some tools that you might be interested in exploring. www.Centerpointe.com is Bill Harris' site. After I spent a few decades practicing meditation, several retreats, and a ton of books, my twin sister, Yvonne, turned me on to Centerpointe's program, which deepened my meditations more than anything else I have tried. It appealed to my inner Dr. Spock as it is an audial input to elicit a

65

particular brain wave. If it sounds interesting, go to the site. Lots of information, and a much more logical explanation than most on the hows of meditation, which will appeal to folks who feel that it is a little too New Age for them. Plus they will send you a free sample CD, called 'The Dive' which is well worth trying. Better living through electronics.

Another lovely toy is www.wilddivine.com. It is a most enjoyable and affordable biofeedback machine that uses a USB connection. There are several levels of a video game that you work through by changing and manipulating your brain waves. Deepak Chopra, Andrew Weil and several other people notable folks were involved in the development, and I love what they came up with.

Recently, a 'Float Spa' opened near me. Back in the seventies, I had a few sessions in a 'sensory deprivation tank' ala John C. Lilly. If you saw William Hurt in 'Altered States' you have an idea of the tank and the procedure. They have an opening price that is reasonable for unlimited use for a month, so off I went. While at Arizona State in 1972, the tank most resembled a coffin, these are fiberglass and resemble an egg. I find this very comforting. It is roomy, with a lid that opens on hydraulics, which does a lot for claustrophobia. You have a light switch, music is piped in, and the water temperature matches the air temperature, which matches your skin temperature. The tank is filled with a dense solution of Magnesium Sulfate, aka Epsom salts. You float- as weightless as an astronaut. I am hooked, so hooked. Not only is it relaxing in the extreme, but you also cannot do anything. Meditating, I know the dishwasher needs to be emptied, but in the tank, it doesn't matter. In that time, I can't do anything but float. The more I do it, the more I have a sense of the monkey mind that nags and chatters constantly simply shutting up. Highly recommended.

An added benefit is the saturation in two minerals that are found only in small amounts in our diet: Magnesium and Sulfur. An abundance of both of these has been shown to support immune system function, ease hypertension and many other things. Dr. Mark Hyman calls Magnesium the most powerful relaxing mineral. When we ingest a magnesium supplement, it has its strongest effect on our digestive system. Since the colon is a muscle, it doesn't take much to relax it, and we have reached 'bowel tolerance' aka diarrhea. But soaking in the magnesium allows our whole system to absorb it, easing the impact. We spent so much of our early millions of years in water, absorption through our skin works very well. Something to think about the next time you read a shampoo label.

Finally, check out www.lumosity.com. These are brain games that get progressively more difficult as you get smarter. There is a lot of information about the science behind it, and I have found it invaluable. Just as I asked you to get up every 45 minutes or so and move around, these games can exercise a different brain function. Like meditation, this helps with focusing on tasks that are challenging, but also it pulls you into your mind, and away from the external world.

One of the most important things to do for health is to disengage. Above are some ways, but just sitting alone, sans phone, computer, and all the things that enmesh us with information constantly, breathing deeply and being grateful is a pleasure that is always available and always renewing.

Clinically, stress is broken into two forms, acute and chronic. Acute stress is what we feel when the driver in front of us slams on his brakes. The adrenalin surge, a sweat, elevated heart rate and blood pressure are all characteristics. This is a good thing, and a necessity for survival. If we hadn't fine tuned it, Neanderthals might be running the world. Chronic stress is a little less benign. This happens when the acute stress happens over and over. Anything can start a chronic stress cycle, from a difficult relationship, to environmental toxins, malnutrition, and negative self-talk or over exercising. Our physiological response is identical, and it is exhausting.

One of the most healing foods ever is a good bone broth. We are used to soups made with canned broth, which is overly salted, and being massed produced, doesn't have the savor, complexity or mineral content of homemade. It isn't difficult to make, but takes time, so make plenty, and freeze some.

Homemade Beef Bone Broth

6 pounds organic beef marrow bones

½ cup raw apple cider vinegar

4 quarts water

3 celery stalks, halved

3 carrots, halved

3 onions, quartered

½ cup fresh parsley

Salt to taste

Put your bones in a large, heavy pot. Add the water and apple cider vinegar, and then let this sit for an hour. The vinegar helps to leach the minerals out of the bones and into the broth. Bring this mixture to a rolling boil and add your veggies. Once the pot comes back to a boil, reduce heat to a simmer, cover and cook for at least 24 hours (some even say up to 72 hours). Check the water levels and stir every few hours. You can always add small amounts of liquid if too much water has cooked off. After cooking, strain the broth. Make sure to inspect the bones for any marrow that may be left behind, and scrape it with a knife into the strained broth. This is an excellent dish by itself, and on an empty stomach, one can experience quite the nutrient rush while drinking this. It has been proven to reduce inflammation, promote healthy hair and nails, stronger bones, and reduced pain levels. You can use it fresh for up to 7 days, and keep it frozen for up to 6 months. It makes a wonderful base for soups!

If you are fifty already and go to the doctor with any regularity, I can guarantee you're being nagged to do a colonoscopy or at least an endoscopy. If you're a woman, you can add a mammogram as well. Both of these tests have inherent dangers, both are covered by insurance, both are being looked at with more skepticism as to their usefulness in early diagnosis (mammograms much more than the colon checks) and both of them are tests for cancer. As I said in the beginning of this book, I am not a doctor, I am not any sort of medical authority. But I have struggled with a lot of health issues and injuries and have come to some conclusions that work well for me.

There is another health problem that many people have, that is exacerbated by being heavy and by getting older. Unless you have managed to avoid the media the last few years, you have heard of sleep apnea. The diagnosis is simple- an overnight sleep test in a lab. A couple of years ago, my husband noticed that I was stopping breathing when I slept. A visit to an ENT doctor, who sent me for a sleep test, revealed that yes, yes I did quit breathing, over 100 times an hour.

Sleep apnea starves your body of oxygen. All of your organs suffer, especially your heart and your brain. But if you die of a heart attack, your death certificate says myocardial infarction, not sleep apnea. I have talked to many people with neurological disorders, and no one ever had a doctor suggest a sleep test. None of my medical care through 6 decades ever said a word about not getting enough sleep. Granted, until I had a serious accident, an annual physical was all I usually did, but if the tests for breast and colon cancer are prophylactic, shouldn't a sleep test be? On my more cynical days, I question why doctors don't start nagging for one on your fiftieth birthday and I am pretty sure that the cancer diagnosis leads to one of the biggest pharmaceutical cash cows, while with sleep apnea? Well, a top of the line CPAP machine is under a thousand dollars. Then maybe they can sell you a couple of filters over the years for a few bucks. I am just saying...

The sleep test itself was daunting. I have talked to many people who have either done them, or who have avoided them because they are anxious about the procedure. Sleep is a mystery. It is the only time many of us are completely alone. It is almost as if we shut a door and disappear. Add to that any sleep issues left over from childhood, and the thought of sleeping in a strange room in a Bride of Frankenstein headdress with a stranger a few feet away who knows more about what is going on than I do was a little, well, off putting.   I did everything I could to avoid it, even asking my doctor to see if fixing my slightly deviated septum solved the problem. Being a good doctor, he refused without the test results. So I made the appointment.

I showed up in the late evening, around 9, with an overnight bag. I even took the pillow I was used to. The room looked like a hotel room. The technician I got was wonderful, comforting, gentle and very low key. There is a lot of attaching of electrodes, maybe twenty five or thirty, which then get bundled over your head, (see Bride of Frankenstein reference above) and plugged into the wall. I had thought this would be disorienting and disturbing, but once I lay down, I hardly noticed it. There was a window on one side of the room that looked into the tech's office, with a curtain pulled closed. Off to sleep I went, more easily than I expected. At the four hour mark, the tech put a CPAP mask on me and left again. The print out that I got showed that I didn't move from then on. I was booted out around six and a week later had my own machine.

I was pretty stoked, I must say, and I could barely wait to get to bed. I got it hooked up, laid down and didn't move for 12 hours, a personal record. Wow. And the dreams were amazing, and two years later, they still are. I am sure the lack of dreaming is a lot of the damage caused by

71

apnea. We apparently don't know a lot about what happens when we sleep, but we do know that a lot of 'processing' goes on in our brains if we dream.   I haven't missed using my CPAP even one a night in two years.

What does this have to do with a detox?   One of my teachers, Reed Davis, with Functional Diagnostic Nutrition, coined the phrase: 'DRESS for success'®.   Diet, Rest, Exercise, Supplementation and Stress Management. Well done, Reed, this covers so much. Sleep and rest are probably the most overlooked aspects of wellness in our culture. Every other aspect of Reed's Big Five get support in our world, but the folks who can supposedly do without sleep are often deified. As long as you are making changes to improve your health, the thirty days of focusing on improving your habits is a perfect time for a sleep hygiene upgrade.

I suggest setting a bedtime, the same every night, and then allowing nine full hours in bed. An hour before you head to bed, or ideally at sunset, either turn off the screens (phone, e-book, computer, television) or check out a program called F.lux. www.justgetflux.com. This is a nifty free app for your computer or phone that will change the blue light they emit to amber. Since watching a cooking show is my favorite thing to do before bed, I invested in amber tinted glasses, but rely on the color change on my computer to alert me that the sun is going down, if I am engrossed. After several million years of sleeping when it gets dark, and waking at dawn, our sleep and wake hormones (melatonin and cortisol respectively) are synchronized with the color of light. I also use a blue light that folks with Seasonal Affective Disorder have found useful. When I was cleaning up my sleep habits, I found that sitting by it for 30 minutes in the morning at the time I wanted to wake up regularly had a wonderful effect on how easily I awoke and how cheerful I could manage to be.

Thanks again, Reed Davis.

Basic Stir Fry technique

1 large Broccoli, cut into florets

¼ Head of Cauliflower, cut into florets

1 large Onion, cut into eighths

1 Cup Chopped Cabbage

2 large Stalks of Celery, diced

6 oz. Mung Bean Sprouts

½ cup Coconut Aminos or Soy Sauce

½ cup Water

¼ cup Coconut Oil

Sriracha to taste

Prep all veggies ahead of time. This is very important, as each one will have a different cooking time, and all of them will cook more quickly than you realize. Make sure you have a large wok or heavy, deep sauté pan. Leave the pan over high heat until very hot. Add the coconut oil, and allow to heat until t shimmers. You will want to start with the cauliflower. Sauté until browned, then reserve to the side. Repeat this step with the broccoli next, and then the celery. Once these veggies are done, sauté the onion until it begins to soften.

Add the cabbage, and just warm it through, as you want it to remain reasonably crispy. At this point, and with the pan still very hot, add the water and aminos and allow to reduce. Add the sriracha paste and the rest of the veggies that are already cooked. Heat everything evenly by tossing the veggies around the pan with two spatulas. Finally add the bean sprouts, toss and remove from the fire. And you're done! Nice and easy...

Another great aspect of this dish is that you can recycle leftovers into it. Make sure to add cook your proteins at the start if you are beginning with raw. Once they are seared and cooked until almost done, remove and put in a bowl nearby so it stays warm. This flavors the sauce and avoids overcooking the meat, chicken or shrimp. Add in the last minute of cooking, along with any other cooked leftovers you like.

Phase Two, Day 16

Wow! Look at the date. You are doing this! By now, along with a good amount of self-righteousness, I hope you are feeling better as well. If you have been following the parameters closely, you are no doubt digesting more efficiently and effectively, sleeping deeply and waking well-rested, and generally finding your energy level and your attitude have improved.   This is the point where I begin to get a little evangelical. People remark that I look good, my eyes and skin are clear, and such, and I love telling them how wonderful this process is. I alienated a few folks the first time, and luckily had friends who cared enough about me to let me know how I came across.

I didn't mean to be disrespectful, but I was. Food and lifestyle choices are about as personal as you can get, and everyone, without exception, has made their own choices based on what works well for them. Whether someone chooses to be a vegan, an athlete, a heroin addict or a bridge player, it is the result of a lifetime of trying things on and either incorporating it into one's life or taking a pass. It is challenging enough to know ourselves, much less someone else.

Which is the point. This is a 'Thirty Day Body Hack.' You picked up this book for your own reasons, but something has you motivated to make some changes. My experience has taught me that people who are open to new things at a point in their life when they can be flexible usually make much better decisions than people who wait until they are forced to make a change. It is always better to quit smoking before you get lung disease.   But it is out of most people's realm to find a part of life that is working okay and see if it can work better.   Maybe it is a good time to reject the old ideas that 'if it ain't broke, don't fix it.' I feel a car metaphor approaching.

Today, when you print out your journal questions, take some time to note what, of all the things you have tried in the last two weeks, is
75

working well. What would you like to incorporate permanently in your routine? What would you like to explore more? If this is just a one time experiment to see how it feels, that's great. But if you want to make a stronger commitment to wellness, here are some thoughts.

1) While this is technically a detoxification regime, since you have eliminated the foods that cause most intolerance reactions, **and** you have reduced your inflammation and toxicity load, it has also functioned as an elimination diet. As you go back to 'normal eating,' keep printing out your journal pages, and go slowly. The foods you have missed the most are very likely to be the ones that your body has a love hate relationship with. I missed coffee tremendously the first time I did this, and found that when I had a cup (on day 31) it wasn't all I remembered. The month away gave me a breather, and now one cup is satisfying. But when I had a couple of bites of a biscuit (I am still a Southerner, it is a birthright thing), I barely had ten minutes before I was in the bathroom. A great indication that biscuits, and more specifically grains, are not my best friends. As you introduce foods back into your meals, since you have gone to all of this effort, go slowly, pay attention and take notes.

2) Decide if you want to be optimally healthy, and what you are willing to do to achieve that goal. Make a commitment, and stick with it. Your health now has taken years to create, and improving it won't happen overnight either. You will get sick- after all; your body has to download the newest virus protection from the Universe. Don't see that as a failure; it is part of the process of being human. And above all, don't confuse being healthy with being thin. A tour of a chemo ward should take care of that delusion, but the media makes certain that the unending deluge of craziness takes a lot of space in our lives. Aspire to optimal health and let your body's intuition guide you. Learn the buzz words your frontal lobes pull out when you are

rationalizing something that you KNOW is not your best choice. (Mine are: 'I deserve, I've earned, just once won't hurt…')

3) Don't use a mistake as a rationalization to give up. I like to think that there is a built in 5% slip up tax. It is easy to skip the gym one day and easier the next. It is also worth the effort to learn to listen to your body; there is no better authority on what you actually need. Learn to trust yourself and be gentle with yourself. It is very similar to raising a child. You need to be patient, and listen carefully, and adore yourself, but also keep the bullshit detector switched on.

4) Find some new friends. We all love people who reinforce our prejudices. If you are committed to health, and need to make changes, it is likely that it is also time to meet some new people. If you were taking up line dancing or trapeze work, it might be difficult to find people already in your circle who could support you and even join you. Take the opportunity to meet some new folks; a yoga class maybe, or a cooking group to minimize meal chores? Get creative, look at what is missing in your life if you are going to maintain your promises to yourself, and go out and find people who will make it easier and more pleasant.

5) Above all, be kind to yourself. One of the most insidious stressors in all of our lives is the negative self-talk. Somewhere along the line, humility got mixed up with self-abuse. And there is nothing in anyone's life as powerful as the narrative we give ourselves, which often has little to do with reality. I realized that every time I stepped out of the shower, I was facing an enormous mirror and every morning thought to myself: 'Good lord, what happened to you?' As per the 'affirmation advocates' I tried telling myself I looked great, but I don't, and knew it. Now, whenever I see myself in a reflective surface, I smile and wave as though I see a dear friend. I realized that my friends and family are beautiful to me in direct proportion to how much I love them, and that my self-critique was me telling

myself that I am unlovable. Not a good thing. (This practice was a little difficult to explain to the woman in the rest room at Threadgill's, but I think she got it...)

Another exercise that I like: Close your eyes and think of someone you love, ideally a child or puppy. A being that you can forgive for anything; someone or something you adore. And the operative word is adore.... Pull up kitten pictures on the Internet if you must, but get that soft eyed, slightly smiling, indulgent expression learned so you can turn it on like a faucet. As soon as you start with the negativity towards yourself, pull out a mirror and put on the face. This is probably my very best stress management technique, not surprising, since calling myself an idiot instead of telling myself I am adorable has been a way of life.

Sauteed Winter Greens

1 large bunch of Kale or Collards, chopped
2 strips of Bacon (optional)
½ an Onion
1 Tbsp. Apple Cider Vinegar
Salt and Pepper to taste

This is a quick and easy side dish without much fuss. Cut bacon into 1/8 inch pieces and brown thoroughly over medium high heat. Add the onions and allow them to soften. Add your chopped greens and sauté them, stirring frequently. Once the greens begin to wilt, add the vinegar and cook until the liquid evaporates. Cook your greens to the texture you like. I always like a bit of crunch, so less is more for me here. You may prefer a more cooked green. This is to your liking. You can even add more protein by topping the greens with a soft fried or poached egg.

Phase Two, Day Seventeen

Every time I go into Half Priced Books, I head towards the diet section. It is always overflowing with books that make an impossible promise: that one specific way of eating will solve all of everyone's problems. Since you are in the midst of an elimination diet, the purpose of which is to flush toxins from your system, as well as give your body a chance to see how it does without foods that frequently cause problems for people, you also know that nutrition and diet are never one size fits all. But the idea that with a simple supplement (pick the buzz of the day, or watch a couple of infomercials) will cause weight loss, muscle gain, smooth skin and stellar teeth with no added effort is seductive, even if our more developed brain knows it is impossible.

I shouldn't have been surprised to learn, at a seminar about the Biotics Research products, that the powers that be often gives supplement manufacturers a several months lead time for 'the next big thing.' If any of the 'big things' actually worked, there wouldn't be a need for a next one would there? But it is a multi million, if not billion dollar market out there. The way most supplements are produced is to shop around, find the lowest bidder, then have the bottles custom labeled, and suddenly this marketing pattern makes sense. If the revolutionary new pill isn't going to work for more than a small percentage of the population, then whether or not it is produced with integrity hardly matters.

One of the real benefits of the detox that you are doing is reminding your body what health feels like. A client will often say to me: 'But Diet Coke doesn't bother me....' Unfortunately, it is the things we do repeatedly, every day, that are likely to be exactly what IS bothering us, but we have become so used to how it makes us feel, that until we take a rest from it for a few weeks, it does seem to have little or no effect. I remember a couple of years ago when I did the first 30 day detox. I was astounded to discover that I was actually a morning person.

We are inundated constantly with ideas and products and images, which end up residing somewhere in our brains. I have always loved Michael Polan's idea, that you should never eat anything you have seen advertised. If a company has spent money devising a way to sell me something, my best guess is that it is something I would not have bought on my own. And the marketing money, often an enormous piece of a budget, was not spent on product quality, of course. Try Polan's idea for a while. You may be surprised how much it limits your options to what you actually need, and how much money it can save you for what truly brings you joy.

Another great thing that occurs in this month is that you become comfortable with standing up for your health. Restaurants in particular have had trouble 'getting' that gluten is a real issue. Often the impact isn't immediately evident and more than one chef I know finds it hard not to be skeptical. When I worked in food service (and I was young, and had a young, bulletproof digestive system), I loathed the folks who asked a ton of questions about the dishes. It felt like they were keeping me from doing my job. But as our food has become more complex and more dangerous, and as reactions to contaminants like preservatives have become more extreme, knowing the food and being able to give accurate information has become a much bigger piece of the job for restaurant people. This is showing up beautifully in many of the newer restaurants who can even reference the farms where the food was grown, and in the upsurge of artisanal restaurants that control the food by making much of it 'in house.'

In taking control of every bite you eat, you have learned a lot of new skills. You have, by now, acquired some mad hunting and gathering knowledge, and probably met some new friends who support your choices along the way. You are getting clearer on reading your body. Now that the chaos of blood sugar spikes and dips is leveling out, you actually know when you are hungry and even better, what it is that you need to refuel with. Cravings often fade as your blood sugar stabilizes, and if green beans are a new obsession, you can trust that they are offering you something you need. And I can eat a bushel of green beans if I can have some butter on them, or maybe a nice walnut oil vinaigrette.

You are also learning to assert yourself to protect your health. Sometime during the last couple of weeks, I am sure you confronted a produce guy or a waitperson about the quality of their offerings, and what you would like to see instead. Even if it was only in your head, make this a lifelong practice. We like to slip into complacency, and not create a stir, and as a result, finding actual food has become difficult. Ask for the sandwich filling on a salad instead of a bun, for the rice noodles on the side with the bowl of Pho, and for the tacos without the shells. When the food industry sees what sells, they always change, so get out there and get visible, and write letters and talk to the people who provide your food. Make me proud.

Tender Greens

1 large bunch of fresh Spinach, cleaned and chopped

3 cloves Garlic, minced

1 Tbsp. Olive Oil

Salt and Pepper to taste

Rinse your spinach well. Heat oil in a heavy sauté pan on medium high heat, and sauté you're garlic until lightly browned. Add the spinach and sauté until it starts to wilt. Promptly remove from the fire as spinach will cook very quickly, and you will want to make sure to pull it from the fire before it throws water. Sautéed spinach can be used as a side dish, or as a stuffing in lettuce wraps with a good protein.

A few chapters ago, I told you that you were going to 'cheat' and that this was not an excuse to give up the detox. You are now past the halfway mark, and before long, you will be out in the real world again. The shakes are a good thing to maintain, if you want an easy and affordable and hyper-healthy meal, and of course, the lemon juice in water to start the day is one of the healthiest things you can do for the rest of your life, but where does everything else fit in? Are you looking at a life without fast food ever again?

It will simply involve trade offs. Imagine a spectrum. At one end is a person who doesn't do any exercise, sits in a desk chair or a car or on a sofa all of the time, eats primarily refined and processed foods, works far too many hours, is engaged with a screen of some sort every working hour, and sleeps badly. We all know him, and many of us have been him. At the other end of the spectrum is a hermit who lives alone in a cave and grows all of his own food, has a pure artesian spring for water and spends the entire day frolicking in the woods and the sunshine. Where you choose to live your life is entirely within your power, and is a choice unique to you. Balance is key, and if your choice is a job that keeps you chained to a desk for hours at a time, then an exercise program is going to be more important to you than it would be for a UPS delivery man, for example. Choosing a frozen pizza for dinner won't be off limits for most of us, occasionally, if it is balanced with some excellent sleeping habits and relaxation. But we get into trouble when we are captured with the adrenalin fueled world that most of us know. In this economy, it feels as though we must constantly push, and look busy and yes, even look stressed, in order to be valued by employers. Certainly many corporations do expect their employees to literally work themselves to death. The medical students I have spoken with lately are a fine example, often being expected to put in one hundred hour weeks. If you think about it, would this be a person you would really choose to make life and death assessments of your health? Yet it is almost a hazing tradition in medical schools.

And for far too many people there are limited options. We are becoming aware of an enormous hunger problem here in the land of plenty. I have been blessed with the means to make a lot of mistakes with my health over the years, and I have enjoyed many of them. But lately, I have been reading a growing mass of research on the health benefits of two things: giving to others, and practicing gratitude. (I gave you a geek alert- if karma/spirituality/and all that nebulous right brain stuff turns you off, skip the rest of the chapter, it isn't written for you Scientific Methodists)

My experience with giving back is this: It forces me to acknowledge that I have more than enough. And the act itself is deeply rewarding. By overvaluing money, we have become a culture of nickel pinchers. It seems that there is little that we share without a price tag on it, either in dollars and cents, time, or service rendered. Once there is a price tag on everything, we lose sight of interdependence; of knowing that just as we took soup next door because we had made a huge pot, if we fall on hard times, there is an investment in whatever we have created as a community. It takes effort to develop a community, and just as it takes a village to raise a child, it takes one to optimize our lives, and thus our health.

Gratitude is another world changer. It runs against the overachiever, because gratitude again means, 'I have enough' or at least that I appreciate what I have and will use it rather than hoard it and spend my days grappling for more. Gratitude slows us. It necessitates slowing down, looking for happiness, and ultimately gratitude is the result.

That addictive, stress-filled, adrenal fired life leads to 'burnout' aka adrenal fatigue. It is a life focused on external stimulation. I would posit that the remedy is simple: more time with one's own thoughts, more decisions based on what is needed, rather than suggested to us by advertisements, more effort to get to know oneself and one's heart and soul. A self-actualized life not only is an end in itself, it will also make you healthier.

End of Right Brain Rant

Broiled Winter Squash

2 lbs of Squash, cut into 1/8 inch rings

2 Tbsp. Coconut Oil

Salt and Pepper to taste

Turn your oven's broiler to high. Peel and prep squash scraping out the seeds, then toss in the coconut oil. Place this into a cast iron skillet and pop under the broiler. Stir every 5 minutes or so, until the squash is browned and cooked to your liking. This is a very quick and delicious side dish for any protein.

Phase Two Chapter 19

According to Ask.com, Americans average a move every five years. I have moved once in the last twenty five and hope to be carried out of here feet first. The inconvenience is overwhelming! And I suspect that is how you are feeling now at the end of your third week of detox. It is inconvenient to find new sources for food, new places you can eat, to establish an exercise routine and worst of all, to clean up your sleep hygiene. The imposition! But remember, you could be moving across the country. As I mentioned yesterday, gratitude enhances health.

But suppose you did have to move. If you got a new job, or retired or decided that time closer to aging parents or grandbabies was important, you would make it happen. The sorts of changes I am proposing are similar to moving to a new town. Pretend the Monday night pizza special is a thousand miles away; what are you going to replace it with? Now is a perfect time to NOT look for another pizza joint. I am a deeply committed hunter and gatherer, (my friend Linda and I have, more than once high fived in a Costco parking lot, while saying: 'And another successful hunting and gathering expedition comes to a close!') but some of my best friends are terrified by food in the rough. You know who you are.

The important realization is this: until you take your power back from the Food-Opolis corporations, you have no control over your health. I firmly believe that once a corporation has stockholders, the integrity of the product is routinely sacrificed for the bottom line. Google a few things… Names for sugar, for example. If the first ingredient listed is sugar, sales will collapse, given the growing realization of how toxic it is. But if you have three different kinds of sugar, they will all be listed lower down. If sugar is something that you are watching, and by now I certainly hope it is, check the number of grams of carbohydrates listed. Also be sure to see what the serving size is. I have seen candy bars that claimed to be four servings, and small bags of potato chips that counted a serving as eight chips. Like that is going to happen.

MSG is another extremely over-used and highly stimulating additive. Technically, it is listed as an 'excitotoxin:' a poison that stimulates. Until I started reading every label, I would have said I wasn't sensitive to it, and the USDA would concur. They claim to have never found evidence that it caused problems for anyone. A very simple way to tell if you are a delicate little thing as I turned out to be is to simply take your pulse before you eat something that you suspect you have sensitivity with. Then take it every half hour for a total of four times. And yes, there are apps on your phone for that, but if you have a heart rate monitor, that makes it very simple. If your pulse goes up more than 6 bpm, you have ingested something your system doesn't like, and it is getting ready for battle. And this is a great stress, that thing we are working so hard to avoid.[1]

Just as you would do if you had moved to a new country, you simply learn the new cuisine. You read the labels, you ask questions, and unless you want to be miserable, you immerse yourself in the culture. The health and nutrition culture is different because there are as many ideas as there are individuals. Again, in a strange country or just a new city, you trust your instincts, your 'gut' feelings, and your sense of direction. For me, grains will always be problematic, but since I realized that before I had become a full blown Celiac (I test negative, but still react to grains) that directs me away from bakeries and pizzerias. But that also lands me in farmers markets and even on farms if I am lucky. Issues with food additives plus a number of years working in restaurants guides me away from most, unless I have researched them well. For many people this would be difficult, and I know that I am very blessed that I love to cook (Grateful!) but avoiding restaurants has made me a better cook. And as more and more of us avoid the restaurants, especially the chain restaurants, the market for locally grown organic food restaurants is booming. We **can** be the change we want to see in the world.

Ultimately, yes, it is a difficult change to make, this eating real food. Tougher for some people than others of course, but it is one of the few things that is universally worthwhile. Demanding nourishing food for everyone is a necessity, if we want to regain our health, and every box of corporate food that isn't bought is a chink in the Big Food monopoly.

[1] For more on this Google 'Coca Pulse Test' or check on my web site for a downloadable chart to keep for three days with a food diary to find food sensitivities. Better yet, buy my earlier book 'A Nutritarian Notebook' from the web site as long as you are there. It has the complete protocol for the Coca Test.

Pan Seared Bok Choy
5 Baby Bok Choy

1 Tbsp. Olive Oil

1 teas. Roasted Sesame Oil

Sesame seeds (garnish)

Wash and trim the bok choy, then cut in half lengthwise. Place in pan cut side down and cook high and fast until the veggies are wilted on top and very brown on the underside. If you prefer the greens more wilted, take the pan off of the Once you reach this point, throw in the sesame oil and remove from the fire. Sprinkle with some sesame seeds to boost the mineral content. Quick and delicious, this makes a great side or addition to any stir-fry or soup.

(This is one of Billie's best dishes, in my humble opinion. I like it as an entrée with some of the roasted mushrooms from an earlier chapter, or even better, with a couple of handfuls of frozen cherries added towards the end. The sweet cherries really enhance the bitterness of the greens, and add antioxidants and anti-inflammatory elements. ED)

Phase Two, Chapter 20

How are you sleeping? Going into the home stretch, have there been changes? The notes that you have so consistently made are going to be invaluable now, as you have been living this life long enough to be seeing some cause and effect. While there are many causes of bad sleep and everyone will have a crappy night once in a while, a major cause is fluctuating blood sugar levels caused by overconsumption of refined carbohydrates. You know now, from experience, that proteins and fats from good sources stabilize your blood sugar levels. Late night eating, in the form of ice cream, crackers or alcohol can crash your blood sugar a few hours later, causing your adrenals to fire and wake you up, urging you to scoot out and run down a rabbit.

If you find that you are awake at 3 or 4, try eating something. Everyone is different, and we all change, so pay attention to the effect of whatever you eat. Protein worked well for me for a long time, in the form of a hardboiled egg or a bite of cheese. If you are avoiding dairy, you might try goat cheese. I believe that most of the problems we have with milk (and I have some) have more to do with it being milk meant for growing a steer rather than a goat. And goats are not 'factory grown' under inhumane conditions and with anti-biotics and hormones nearly as much as cows are in this country. Small batch goat cheese makers are proliferating, and if you are in Austin, I recommend Pure Luck. Drive out to Dripping Springs and meet your source!

Try a slow absorption carbohydrate if you don't get good results from protein. The closer to your bedside you have it, the less you will waken to grab it, so dried fruit or a few nuts are a possibility. If you continue to journal about your health, you will quickly find something that works.

Another option is a product from Biotics Research, called Glucobalance.® Developed by Dr. Jonathan Wright, a Harvard trained physician and researcher in Natural Medicine, it is made up of a number of key nutrients (remember that Biotics products are sourced from food) including Niacin and Niacinimide that support healthy blood sugar balance on a cellular level. There is documentation and research spanning years both in Europe and the United States on this product. It is also full of trace minerals that are difficult to find in the modern diet. Doubtless a more complete snack than that bunny your adrenals wanted you to go run down. And although the efficacy of this product has been well researched and documented, 'These statements have not been evaluated by the FDA and are not intended to diagnose, cure, prevent or treat any disease.' Given that the FDA has approved so many things that compromise my health, I have to wonder what that statement even means….

Temperature, dark and noise are also massive sleep disruptors. Find what works for you. I know that as people are together over time, ideal sleep conditions can change, but tweak everything until you can both get a solid night's sleep. Anything that improves everything we do in bed has to be worthwhile, right?

And remember the discussion about turning off the screens an hour before bed time? I was serious about that. The blue light from the screens (yes, all of them, telephone, computer and television, and more) stimulates cortisol, aka the stress hormone. In fact, it is more of a waking up hormone, stimulated by the bluish light at dawn. For millions of years, we went to sleep when the lights went out, and sunset is an amber colored light which signals our bodies to produce melatonin. Given the light pollution that we are exposed to constantly, no wonder 'sleep aids' are seeing record sales.

My easy and cheap solution was a pair of amber tinted glasses for use after dark. They have made a big difference in how easily I can get to sleep and the depth of my sleep once I drop off.

Beet, Green Bean and Red Onion Salad

2 large Beets, peeled and roasted

1 lb Green Beans, blanched

½ Red Onion, sliced thin

3 Tbsp. Olive Oil

2 tsp. Red Wine Vinegar

½ cup toasted walnuts

¼ lb. Feta (optional)

Salt and Pepper to

Scrub your beets well to remove dirt. (A friend runs hers in the dishwasher when she doesn't have a full load, and swears by the method.) Wrap in foil, and place in a sheet pan. Beets should roast in a 400 degree oven for 30 minutes until tender. This will vary greatly with the size of the beets, so test by sticking with the tip of a paring knife. You want a little resistance. Cool them while you prep the rest of the salad.

Blanch the green beans in boiling water for 3 minutes. Remove and place in an ice water bath to stop them from cooking. This also helps them to retain their beautiful green color and keeps them crispy. Peel the beets if you like, or just trim, and cut into bite sized chunks. Add the green beans, onions, vinegar and olive oil and taste for salt and pepper. I like it with much more freshly ground pepper than you would think. Add the feta and/or walnuts if you like.

Phase Two, Chapter 21

Until a very few years ago, most of our days were spent doing steady rhythmic movements. Scything grain, sewing, stirring pots, walking, rocking babies, all created a cadence in our bodies. About four times a year, I feel an urge to get to the Gulf, and sit for an hour or several hours, as though the rhythm of the waves somehow re-calibrates me. This seems to happen more often in the sedentary winter months, and the times when I don't swim as much. While exercise, seen as a half hour or so at the gym three times a week, may be a fine thing, I have come to believe that movement is more valuable. The current buzzword is: 'Sitting is the cigarettes of the 21st century.' Locked to a computer screen may not be the healthiest way to spend our days, yet that is precisely what most of us do. Posterior proliferation is the most obvious symptom, and limited circulation, as well as postural problems and organ problems because people simply are not engineered to sit for long periods. A midday aerobics class is fine, but I believe that the tempo of our bodies needs to be wound like a watch.

We see exercise as good because it 'burns calories.' When I began this journey, the first words Dr. Marlene Merritt said to me were: 'I guess you've discovered that 'calories in and calories out' doesn't work....' True, and in particular for post-menopausal ladies who have descended from a long, long line of famine survivors. I believe we may be a majority in this country soon. Certainly the metabolic fires can be helped along with cardio, but, as with nutrition, you can find a million theories of exercise, mostly contradictory. Discovering what works well for you is a lifelong challenge. It is tempting to just buy the next new thing, which may well work, either in the short term or for some segment of the population. It is similar to seeing an ad for a new antidepressant drug and having your doctor write a prescription because even with side effects, maybe you will be happier. Or you can look inside and maybe discover why you aren't as happy as you would like to be and fix that.   The second option sounds a little more empowering, doesn't it?

Historically, the struggle has been to find enough calories to fuel us doing the daily necessities. Efficiency is a good thing, and because of past food scarcity, laziness became a survival skill. Digestion is one of the biggest users of energy in our bodies, second only to our enormous brains (20% of energy for brains regardless of whether you are reading String Theory or on Facebook, and roughly 10-12% for digestion.) Refined foods are much less calorically expensive to break down and absorb, and refined carbohydrates are especially cheap, breaking down with amylase, found in saliva. For a complex carbohydrate source, like an apple, this is the beginning of digestion. The simpler the starch and sugar that needs to be broken down, the faster it goes into the blood stream. It would be interesting to see a race between drinking a HFCS soda and injecting glucose into a vein. I'm not sure which horse I would bet on.

For decades, we have focused on the caloric count as the value of food. The result has been a populace willing to buy 'empty food.' Real food, nutritious food, will naturally be caloric. The next time you are at your grocery, watch for 'new, improved, low calorie' products and check out the rather frightening list of ingredients.

We are finally, in the last few years, acknowledging the fat scam that has made us phobic of many of the most nutritionally dense foods. Studies from the UK recently are dispelling the saturated fat as killer food lies that have in fact made us sicker and deader and fatter. The butter isn't destroying your arteries, it's the sugar. And it is also hammering your metabolism. Here are results of a USDA study done in 1998, when our tribal superstition was still anti-saturated fats.

92

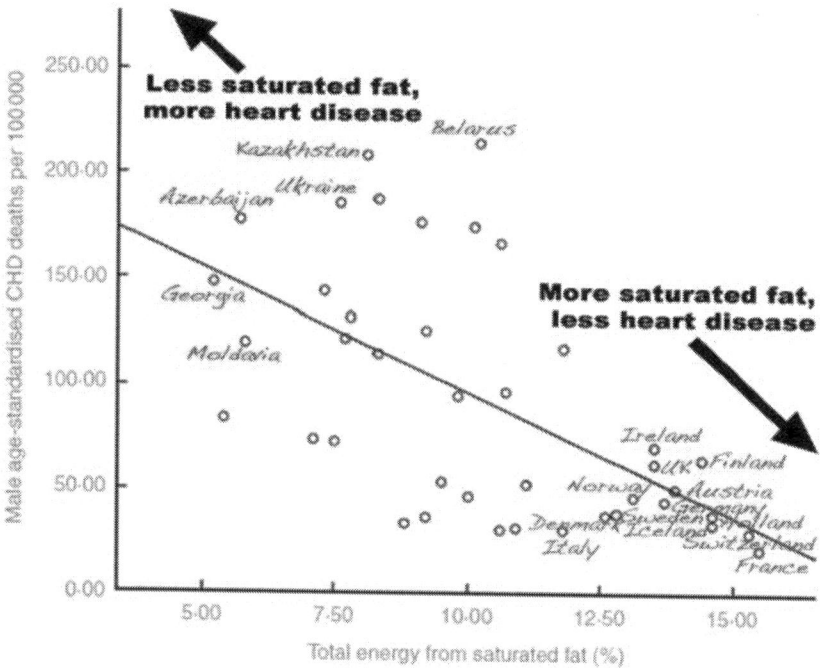

Fig. 1. Saturated fat intake and CHD mortality in Europe (1998). R^2 inear = 0.339.

It's not the quantity of the fats in our diet that is killing us, it is the quality of the fats. I have read repeatedly that consumption of meat leads to early death. I believe there are two factors working here. We have gotten spoiled by the government subsidy of grains, providing cheap livestock feed. The grains do the same thing to other animals that they do for us; they give us the ability to pile on that lifesaving belly fat that we can access in a famine. Cattle are raised in feed lots, where the septic conditions are so dreadful that shovelfuls of antibiotics per animal are needed to at least keep them breathing, if not healthy. The grain fermentation in feed lots has created stupendous quantities of methane, which, with grass fed animals is much less, and is well dispersed. But the grains had another effect- they changed the chemistries in the animals stomachs, creating an excellent host for bugs like Escherichia-coli, aka e-coli. Toss in some antibiotics and you are on your way to bacteria the size of Chihuahuas and about as aggressive.

93

For the sake of the planet, sustainability and plain old Karma, we must all stop supporting the factory farming of animals.

Chicken Curry

4 Boneless Skinless Chicken Breasts

2 Quarts chicken broth or stock

12oz. Can Coconut Milk

2 Tbsp. Curry Powder

4 Baby Bok Choy, washed and coarse chopped

Salt to taste

In a large saucepan, heat the broth over medium heat to just a simmer. Poach the chicken breasts in the broth for 30 minutes or until done through. (160°) Set them aside and add the curry powder and the coconut milk to the broth. Cook over medium high heat until this reduces by a third, about 45 minutes or so. Once your broth is reduced, shred the chicken breasts and add them back into the liquid. Add the bok choy and cook for another 20 minutes. Remove the dish from the heat and add the mung bean sprouts. Enjoy this warm and hearty dish on a good cold day!

Phase Two Chapter 22

A traditionally normal carbohydrate diet now known as a 'low carbohydrate diet' is what our bodies, with a spectrum of variations, are best at digesting. When the refined foods became hugely profitable, the marketing of 'convenience foods' mushroomed. Supposed food experts extol the virtues of these foods, but we did exceedingly well for millennia without them. Our natural (and evolutionarily advantageous) laziness made these exquisitely seductive, and with more women going to work outside the home and more people staying single home cooking all but disappeared. Our intake of simple starches and sugars went through the ceiling, and our stomachs suppressed the manufacture of HCl, necessary to break down protein. www.westonaprice.org/thumbs-up-reviews/why-stomach-acid-is-good-for-you-by-jonathan-wright-and-lane-lenard is a PDF describing why this is dangerous. Like the cattle eating grains, the suppressed acid has calamitous effects on our digestion, from one end to the other.

This is one of the reasons that this detox starts with a big dose of enzymes. Food manufacturers love big eaters, and one way to attract these folks is to 'process' the food until it is texturally maximized for ease of eating and digestion. Sounds like a good thing, right? Not so much. This process creates something akin to baby food. Until the last century, meat was pretty tough, fruits and vegetables had much more fiber before they were bred to ripen at the same size, same time and become inflated with carbohydrates. Gathering and preparing food was everyone's primary occupation, and was a full time job. Chewing and digestion was a lot of work. To suddenly move from that diet, established over millennia, to drinking a lot of our calories in nutritionally negative sodas and juices, and eating food that is effectively pre-chewed, put a lot of our digestive abilities to sleep if not a coma. We also moved from eating saturated fats like lard and butter to oils such as soy and canola. Our carbohydrate intake soared, making food manufacturing/processing highly profitable. If dinner became macaroni and cheese from a box, the farmers, growing green beans and peppers and tomatoes necessarily found other work, selling their land to corporate farming.

The cost in terms of health has been brutal. Which, along with the enrichment of corporate agriculture made a lot of pharmaceutical manufacturers wealthy? I do love a nice conspiracy theory, don't you? On a personal level, this also reduced the need for our state of the art digestive system. When food is meager, it is important to be able to break down and get nourishment from a variety of sources. This gave us the carnivore stomach, where protein is turned to a paste called *chyme* by a hydrochloric acid level of 1.5 to 3.0. If you own a television, you have no doubt heard a lot of brainwashing about the need to lower stomach acid. If you followed the link above (highly recommended) you know that acid reflux is caused by the food in the stomach not being broken down, putrifying, creating gas which is then belched through what is ideally a one way valve, and into the esophagus. While lowering the acidity can reduce the acid reflux, it isn't doing your nutrition or your body in general any favors.

Good digestion isn't the only advantage of normalizing stomach acid. The high acid also acts as our best defense against ingesting pathogens. Remember how the cattle being fed grain supported the proliferation of *e. coli*?[1] Hmmm. The use of massive antibiotics in feed lots has allowed these bacteria to create defenses, becoming more antibiotic resistant, in much the same way that salmonella did. Yet Dr. Susan Sumner, a food scientist from Virginia Polytechnic Institute has found that two separate spray bottles, one of hydrogen peroxide and one of white vinegar, applied to produce. Use two separate bottles, and don't mix them! You will create paracetic acid, potentially harmful and also ineffective in reducing pathogens eliminated heavy infestations of e.coli, salmonella and shigella more effectively than chlorine bleach. [2] With commercial vinegar acidity at 2.5 to 3.4, reducing stomach acid makes even less sense, doesn't it?

To learn more about stomach acid go to my web site, www.austin-nutritional-therapy.com or pick up Dr. Jonathan Wright's book, 'Why Stomach Acid is Good For You.'

1 'The End of Food' Paul Roberts, 2009
2 'Science News' August 8, 1998

Lentils– Cold Salad or Lettuce wrap

1 lb. Lentils, sprouted and rinsed
1 large Onion
3 cloves Garlic, minced
1/4 cup Olive Oil
Salt and Pepper to taste

Sprout your lentils by rinsing the dried beans, allowing them to sit in cold fresh water for 6 to 8 hours, then pour off into a colander or strainer and rinse in fresh water several times a day until you see small sprouts starting from the beans, and the skins have broken open. Place the beans in a heavy pot and fill with water about 1/2 inch over the top of the lentils. Add the onion and garlic, and cook covered over medium-low heat until the lentils are tender, about 30 minutes. Uncover and add the olive oil, cooking the lentils until they are creamy and tender. This dish can be eaten hot over kelp noodles, or cold on top of a salad or in a lettuce wrap. Add some of the spinach you already cooked.

Phase Two, Chapter 23

Remember health class? It often occurred around seventh grade, when 'changes in your body' began to appear. Now, with the ready availability of food and thus young women with plenty of fat to make estrogen, and support a pregnancy, our bodies are doing exactly what they were developed to do: crank out some babies ASAP while food is abundant and the likelihood of survival is greatest. In 1900, girls reached puberty at around fifteen, and in 1990, the age had dropped to twelve and a half. A fine argument could be made for health education starting a lot earlier, perhaps? And another argument could be made for health education, starting perhaps in third grade, including basics of digestion and nutrition. Most of the people I get into nutrition discussions with know where food goes in and poop comes out, but the process in between is a mystery. If we want to optimize well-being we must each take responsibility for our health. Our cultural paradigm for this is to wait until we are actually ill and then go to a doctor for a prescription. Each of us is the best source of information on our selves, and education to de-mystify the processes that constantly engage us will make that information so much more available. {{Kicking away that pesky soap box}}

Yesterday, I think we had gotten a meal as far as your stomach, and the extreme acidity there. This is important to break down protein, and to kill pathogens. Our stomach lining is most functional and prepared to absorb nutrients when bathed in acid. And just as the bad bugs are decimated by acid, the good bugs, necessary for so many body functions and processes, are delighted with high acidity. It is tempting to think of our organs performing only one function, but in fact, they are multi-tasking constantly. The support system for many of these complex processes is the microorganisms that outnumber our cells by a factor of 10 to 1. What makes these little fellows happy is the same thing that makes us happy: good food, a warm comfortable place to live and

98

something to do. They love soluble fiber, and ferment it, which benefits us by breaking down foods for us to assimilate. But there is an enormous variety of gut microbes, some wonderfully adapted to work symbiotically with us, some not so much. A lot of these less desirable folks can be dealt with in the stomach, but once they get to your gut, if they like the environment, they can settle in and create all sorts of havoc.

In 1908, Elle Metchnikoff, a Russian researcher, received the Nobel Prize for his studies on gut flora and his theory that the bad guys could be crowded out by adding in good guys. He also believed that aging was a result of less than adequate digestion allowing food to putrify in the gut, creating toxins that were then absorbed, and here we are back to low stomach acid once more. The probiotics and fermented foods that Metchnikoff recommended have been used for centuries. If you go to a Korean restaurant, you will get Kimchee, and a deli gives you a pickle. Now we also have available capsules and liquid forms of probiotics. In Phase Three you will be using Bio-Doph 7 to reseed the flora in your own gut.

I would like for you to think of your gut as a neighborhood. You will have some homeowners, as well as some renters. In fact the majority of your population will be migrant workers who stay for a while, do some chores and move on. If you were blessed with a mother who nursed you for several weeks, you may also have some additional populations that are relatively permanent. It is a fine idea to make the gut ambiance as welcoming as you can for the desirable folks. Stomach acid helps them survive into your digestive system. Soluble fiber, like psyllium seed husks and lots of fruits and vegetables make them very happy.

The United States, perhaps due to the miraculous antibiotic revolution, has become germ phobic. We have bottles of antibacterial soaps and washes posted outside grocery stores, antibacterial wipes everywhere, and these are definitely the enemies of your gut flora. If you don't believe that you absorb everything that touches your skin, try rubbing a piece of cut garlic on your foot and see how quickly you taste it. If you pay attention while washing your hair, you will notice a faint taste of soap in your mouth very quickly. Understandably, when the flu bugs seem to be everywhere, it is tempting to just obliterate everything, but much of your immune system is fostered in your intestines. Over use of anti bacterials can destroy much of what you are trying hard to support. It makes more sense to trust your immune system to do its job than it does to eradicate everything, and to do what you can to keep it in top condition.

Another final piece of good digestion is hydration. Often, things like constipation, weakness and even heart palpitations are symptoms of dehydration. The accepted thinking is that we need to divide body weight by 2 and the result is the number of ounces of water we need to be taking in. I would increase that by a good margin if you are overheating, or drink anything like caffeinated beverages or alcohol that are diuretics. Your body is made up mostly of water and needs replenishment to function well. And of course, water is necessary for eliminating wastes. Imagine that you have swept your whole house, and then leave the pile of dust on the floor. It will quickly disperse. In the same way, without enough water all the cleaning your body can manage may be wasted if there is not enough water to flush things out and keep them from being re-absorbed.

Back on Day 5, I mentioned lectins. Before Monsanto, plants developed their own protection from insects and other predators. These are proteins that can bind to carbohydrates and act as anti-fungals and insecticides. Since they also have a strong bitter taste, they also discourage grazing animals. They are most abundant as the seed matures.

Lectins are found in grains, particularly grains high in gluten. As botanical engineers bred grains with higher and higher protein levels,

100

the toxins also increased. They are often spliced into GMO foods to enhance resistance.[1] Lectins are also found in the nightshade vegetables like tomatoes, potatoes, eggplant and peppers. People with joint pain can often get relief by avoiding these foods. Tree nuts have lectins. Dairy is another source, if the source cows are fed grains rather than being pastured, and finally legumes are perhaps the highest source in most diets.

Ancient cultures found many ways to reduce the lectins in foods. When you have no food to waste, a cook can become very inventive. Fermentation, soaking and sprouting can all significantly lower lectin levels. Your grandmother wasn't just saving fuel by soaking her beans; she was also washing away the natural poisons. In the lentil recipe, you read instructions for soaking legumes and sprouting them. (And during the initial soak, I like to add liquid minerals to the soak water, which enhances the nutritional value greatly.) This also transforms a dried and starchy bean into a nascent plant, lowering the carbohydrates as the embryonic seedling consumes the starch. All good stuff!

Sprouting is fine for all cooked beans, but they still need to be thoroughly cooked. The larger beans, and red kidney beans in particular, can be toxic if eaten raw or even undercooked. For this reason I don't like using a slow cooker for beans. For this black bean preparation, I soak the beans overnight, rinse them well, and then let them air dry for a couple of hours before cooking.

And lectins aren't all bad. They appear to inhibit the growth of bacteria, viruses, fungi, and perhaps even cancer cells. But everyone has a different level for too much of a good thing, and this elimination diet is a fine way to find your own susceptibilities. If you routinely consume any of the lectin bearing foods, try cutting them out for 30 days and then add in one at a time. This is where I differ with the Classic Paleonistas. Legumes have so much wonderful nutrition, including fiber, vitamins and if well prepared, an abundance of minerals and good

101

protein, that it is in almost everyone's interest to eat them regularly.

1. Rhodes, Jonathan M.   Genetically modified foods and the Pusztai affair. BMJ. May 8, 1999

Black Bean Soup Cubana

1 pound black turtle beans, soaked and rinsed

1 Tablespoon ground cumin

1 Tablespoon dried oregano

Dried red pepper flakes

1 cup chopped peppers*

1 cup chopped yellow onion

6 cloves garlic, chopped

Olive oil for sautéing

¼ cup lime juice

1 Tablespoon honey

Salt and pepper to taste

In a large stockpot, place the beans, cumin, oregano and pepper flakes. Cover with water to one inch over the beans and either simmer on top of the stove or place in a 225° oven for 45 minutes to an hour, until tender stirring and adding water as needed.

In a skillet, heat enough oil to cover the bottom of the pan. Add the onions and peppers and cook gently until translucent. Add the garlic and cook just until you can smell it cooking. Puree in a food processor or blender. ** Add to the beans along with the honey and lime juice, and return to the oven or simmer for another 45 minutes.

Garnish with chopped onion, or cilantro, crumbled cotija cheese, avocado slices... A spoonful of dry sherry stirred in before serving is also traditional.

* The variety of peppers is what makes this soup. You can use all sweet bell peppers, or maybe a chipotle or even some pickled pepperoncini. Use your imagination.

** This is a *sofrito*. It is a basic in many Latin American dishes, and can be made in bulk. I make a lot at once, and freeze it in 8 oz. containers. It is instantly a soup base but can also be used to season taco meat, or as a braising liquid.

From an earlier chapter, I hope you got that the source of stress is how you engage with the world. This is clearly something that you are in charge of, so why are we exhausting ourselves? Well, because it feels so good! Stress isn't our enemy, but like many good things, it is easy to overdo. Because our hardwiring keeps us constantly looking for food, if we are hungry or malnourished, our nervous system will keep us looking for the next meal, which opens us to the sensual world. It is stimulating and thrilling and it interconnects us. Given the state of the Standard American Diet and the epidemic of malnutrition, perhaps it is not so surprising that we have such a strong urge to stay connected.

Most clients, when changing their diets for the better and particularly when they do a detox program, comment that they are suddenly happier. Certainly having the building blocks for hormones is a contributor, but I have come to believe that when we optimize our nourishment, we are calmed on the hunger front, and more able to relax and check in with the balance of the external world, and our own internal lives.

One of the real downside hazards of our proliferating information funnel is how seductively it can keep us bound to what the media wants us to hear and believe, letting our trust in our own innate wisdom languish. The entire WMD kerfuffle is a good example, and the Cholesterol Con is another. Now we are looking at Western Medicine, and the pharmaceutical corporations as well as behemoths like the food and petroleum lobbies, and personally, they sure feel a lot like a kerfuffle to me.

Something I would like you to do- go into your pantry and find a bottle or box with a 'nutrition label.' You will notice that on the right side of the label, protein, fat and carbs as well as vitamins and minerals have a listing as a % of the daily requirement. A few years back, most countries

104

set an upper limit of 10% of calories from sugar, and our 1992 update of the Food Pyramid was based on this. The sugar industry went nuts, and if you look at the nutrition label, you will note that there is not a listing for a daily requirement for sugar. Ten percent, or about 25 grams of sugar a day, would be one banana and a spoonful of honey in your morning coffee; or an 8 ounce Coca Cola.

One of the dangers is that this addresses only fructose. The starches in a food will be listed as carbohydrates, but with refined carbs, the glycemic index, or rate at which the calories hit the blood stream can be even faster than sugars. www.health.harvard.edu lists the glycemic index for a plain white baguette as 95, a Coca Cola at 63, oatmeal at 66 and premium ice cream at 38. This is starting to look a little like a WMD, isn't it?

From the pre-recorded 'news' we are fed, often on the 'breakthroughs in medication' to the recommendation by the USDA to get recommending 6-11 servings of grains as the basis for a healthy diet, to Wal-Mart going organic and Coca Cola's anti-obesity campaign, the quality of information parallels the quality of our food. There is good, nutritious food available, but you have to find it buried under a lot of 'food like substances.' In the same way, there is solid information on how we can optimize our health, rather than stay just above the edge of 'not sick.' This is where the inner connection comes in. We have been brainwashed to be Scientific Methodists: If there is a study that 'proves' a theory, and it is published, it is true. But as we are finding, most food studies are funded by Big Food interests; it is difficult to find anything about agriculture that isn't paid for by Monsanto. Even when a study appears to be objective, it is astoundingly easy to falsify or misrepresent the results. Very often with pharmaceutical testing, the negative results simply do not get reported. And every drug that the FDA has recalled, they initially approved. One might think that before something is approved, more research might be in order?

I think the real litmus for all of us must be our knowledge, our ability to research for ourselves, and our intuition. Because of the overwhelming amount of knowledge out there, we will take shortcuts, inevitably. I am not going to bone up on internal combustion engines, but instead have mechanics that I trust. I am blessed to be married to one of them and mother to the other one. If we choose to have a meal away from our kitchens, we are trusting the cook, the servers, the suppliers, the dishwashers and everyone who has touched our food since it was a seed to have our best interests and our health as a priority. And to live on minimum wage.

Western Medicine has made great strides, and as I have said repeatedly, I am hugely grateful to my orthopedic surgeon's mom for pushing him through medical school. I can walk, and without his expertise I would still be in a wheelchair. It also has a lot to answer for. I recently watched an ad for a medication for managing 'non-mitral valve fibrillation.' It included the usual side effects, from nausea to death. www.healthline.com lists dehydration as a common cause of atrial fibrillation, particularly with elderly people. The ad never mentioned: 'Drink a glass of water and see if that helps.' I don't think pill ads are who I want to trust with my health, yet the continuing education required of doctors to maintain their licenses (in Texas, 48 hours every 2 years, 2 of which must involve medical ethics, and responsibility and 24 of which can be 'informal study') are funded almost exclusively by pharmaceutical companies.

Ultimately, I don't want to treat a symptom, I want to treat the underlying cause. My experience (and the good old innate wisdom) has indicated that for me, managing my stress, giving my body the best available nourishment, exercising and prioritizing rest and sleep is the most effective program I can use to optimize my health without ever needing to know what the underlying cause of the symptom was in many situations. It is trusting ourselves rather than blindly believing an idea because it was in the news that supports us finding the sweet spot.

106

As Abraham Lincoln is quoted saying: 'Just because it was on the Internet doesn't mean it is true.'

Any list of 'The ten healthiest foods' will include a lot of greens. Here is another way to cook them which even kids seem to love. I don't need to reiterate the importance of buying organic, hopefully from the hands that harvested that morning, do I?

Confederate Choucroute

1 head of green cabbage (I like the Savoy)

1 bunch collards, de-stemmed

3 Tart apples (Granny Smith, Pippin, Melrose…)

½ cup dry white wine or vermouth (optional)

1 Tablespoon honey

¼ cup cider vinegar

¼ cup coarse mustard

Salt and pepper

Put everything in a slow cooker or a lidded casserole and toss well to mix. There should be plenty of moisture, but keep an eye on it. Cook on low for 5-6 hours or in the oven at 200°, covered.

Protein can be added to this, if you like, from a handful of chopped ham to pork chops to sausage. Just make sure the meat stays covered by the vegetables and be vigilant with the moisture level. Very nice with more mustard on the side and maybe a little horseradish?

Phase Three, Chapter 25

Ahh, what an amazing achievement! Twenty five days away from most of the foods that make up the Standard American Diet, achieving unheard of hunting and gathering skills, and empowering yourself in the kitchen has had a wonderful effect, hasn't it? Empowerment really is the point of this exercise. We all make the decision for ourselves on what we will delegate to experts and what we will take responsibility for. There is tremendous support for convenience, but it is coming at greater cost. After this month, you will have a knowledge of self-care that will help you for the rest of your life!

This is the best part of the detox program to me. It addresses cell malnourishment and joint damage, and it feels great! It is important to follow this guide as closely as possible through each phase. If Biotics Research products are not available to you, these descriptions can help you find substitutes. Check www.bioticsresearch.com for more information. Your approved food list can be eaten in any combination, but it is important to rotate different foods in, especially the proteins. You will continue the two meals from these foods and the twice daily shakes. You will also add:

Optimal EFAs- a combination of fish, flax and borage oils to provide a spectrum of Essential Fatty Acids. (Vegetarians can use a source such as Black Currant seed oil, available from Biotic's Research) 2 gel caps, 3 times a day. These are exactly what they say they are- ESSENTIAL Fatty Acids. The low fat diet that most of us tried to follow in the past 40 years has done some serious damage to our health. While it may well be an improvement over the rancid seed oils that we were hoodwinked into eating, we have only to compare the rates of heart disease, stroke, cancer and other dangerous health threats to our consumption of these oils and our elimination of the life-enhancing fish, coconut, butter and other traditional sources of fat to realize that we have been duped. I encourage you to find Sally Fallon Morel's 'The Oiling of America' on YouTube and invest an hour of your time watching it. Then clean out your pantry.

Pro-multi plus- A predominately food based*, high potency multivitamin/mineral. 1-2 caps, 3 times a day. This is a wonderfully complete multiple vitamin and mineral supplement. 6 capsules seem like a lot, but almost everything in those capsules is food. The herbs in particular (all organic) take a lot of room, but being made from food, our bodies can recognize and absorb the nutrients. This has been my 'go-to' basic supplement for anyone, and I am in my fourth year of using it, still delighted with the results. This product is especially useful in normalizing sugar metabolism.

It is important to note here that the USDA analysis of nutrition in foods was last done in the fifties. There has been a great deal of resistance to reassessing the foods we eat. When the figures you find for example, for the amount of Vitamin C in an orange were done prior to the use of most chemical fertilizers, and certainly before foods were often transported and held for days or weeks before eating, they don't reflect reality. Just as we need vitamins and minerals to survive, a plant or animal needs similar nutrition. Modern agricultural methods, especially monocropping, have exhausted much of our soil, and chemicals like ammonium nitrate have become the standard for 'fertilizer.' As the name implies, it is NH_4NO_3 and nothing else. When we don't return the compost and manure to the soil the minerals cannot exist in the food. Just as we don't do well with low minerals, other organisms don't do well either, and making the vitamins that are needed for them to thrive is difficult to impossible and so are in much lower concentrations than the idealized numbers from decades past. If the subject interests you, I highly recommend a film, 'King Corn' from 2007, available from Netflix. www.kingcorn.net

Bio-Doph-7 Plus- a rich variety of probiotics for GI repair. 1-2 tablets, once daily. Since you have been busily cleaning house for weeks, your gut is much cleaner, and as we are learning, clean and health may not be synonymous. This is a wonderful source for the lovely little bugs that we want proliferating to help us digest, but just as importantly, to help make many of the vitamins, hormones and other elements that keep us happy and healthy. The good guys, in sufficient numbers, are instrumental in crowding out the bad guys, and since you have been detoxing, there is a lot of real estate available there. It is important to get the population established, and this is a wonderful source for the living microbiota as well as prebiotics, which the probiotics feed on. Essentially you are offering a buffet for the newcomers; how hospitable.

Chondrosamine Plus- a broad spectrum joint repair product. 1-2 tablets, three times a day. Chondrosamine alone has been demonstrated to help collagen function in joints. This compound also contains Niacin, Vitamin C, folic acid, pantothenic acid and manganese, all of which are stripped from our food during processing. These are also necessary to support the action of the Chondrosamine, as well as being powerfully anti-inflammatory and destroyers of free radicals. Not appropriate for vegetarians, as the source is bovine.

If joint issues are a problem, you might consider adding collagen to your shakes as you rebuild. My preference is Great Lakes brand, available from my web site. www.austin-nutritional-therapy.com.

Bio-D-Emulsion Forte- Emulsified Vit D3. 2000 IU per drop. 1-2 drops twice daily. Vitamin D has been much in the news lately, and there seems to be an epidemic of low Vitamin D levels, which can lead to all sorts of trouble, from thyroid problems to osteoporosis and more. This is a drop, making it very easy to use and absorb, and is also quite inexpensive, roughly 2$ a month. An indoor lifestyle and the use of sunscreens are thought to be primary causes of the widespread *Hypovitaminosis D.*

KappArrest- NF-kappaB inhibitor to reduce inflammation. 3 capsules twice a day. I use this every day for inflammation and find it quite effective. It has turmeric, boswella, ginger and green tea among other things, and works by down regulating the inflammatory pathways. This means that it doesn't interfere with your body's own anti-inflammatory functions in the way that NSAIDs can.

This should give you a good idea of what you are rebuilding. You will be taking in larger than usual amounts for a few days, and as I said earlier, this is my favorite part of the detox because it just feels so good!

*The K-1 is unstable if it is food sourced, and if you want to get Vitamin K from a food, the best source is natto. Google it. I won't be eating the natto.

Since you are adding a variety of probiotics back into your tummy, now is a good time to learn about miso. This is a fermented paste used often in Asian cooking. Made from soybeans or other grains, this belies the usual prohibition, because fermentation not only breaks down the proteins, making them easily assimilable, but also remains in the miso itself with enormous benefits for our digestion. It also is a source of all of the amino acids, making it particularly beneficial for vegetarians. They are also abundant in enzymes and probiotics.

Very generally, lighter misos have a gentler, perhaps less complex flavor. The taste may be acquired, and caution is advised, as the flavor can be overwhelmingly salty. Probably the most common use of miso in the United States is in soup.

Basic Miso Soup

4   cups water

¼-1/3 cup miso paste

3 chopped green onions

1" piece of *kombu** and/or shredded *nori**

Roasted sesame oil

If you are using one of the seaweeds, simmer gently in the water for 5-10 minutes. This will eliminate much of the 'fishy flavor, and maximize the release of the minerals into the soup. Add the miso, and stir well, cooking over very low heat to preserve the probiotics. Serve hot with the green onion and sesame oil to garnish.

Of course, this is just the beginning. I love leftover greens in miso soup, and shreds of chicken, pork or even a few shrimp are lovely. It can also be a base for any pureed soup, once the seaweed is strained out, leaving its mineral content behind. Tofu is traditional, and if you tolerate soy, go for it.

Kombu and *nori* are two of the more common dried seaweeds, now widely available. They are mineral rich, and add a deep umami flavor to anything cooked with liquid. A nice piece of *kombu* was my secret ingredient in chili for years, pulled out just before serving. Highly recommended also in any bone broth or soup.

Back when we started this, I mentioned Reed Davis' mantra: DRESS®: Diet, Rest, Exercise, Stress Management and Supplementation. I have rather glossed over the exercise piece of it, because with all the changes, and yes, stresses, instituting an exercise regime can be too much. But while you are still in change mode, and especially now when you are feeling great, it is something to think about.

Exercise wasn't recommended for weight loss until the fifties, when one of my personal idols, Jack Lalanne and television created a perfect storm and fitness became fashionable. He is often called the Godfather of Fitness. But my favorite autobiographical story was his report of being a 'sugarholic' and describing himself as 'a miserable god damn kid; it was hell.' He was a high school dropout and bulimic He turned his life around after hearing a lecture on nutrition by another nutrition pioneer, Paul Bragg. He was fifteen years old, so that would have been 1929.

Lalanne was known as a bodybuilder and exercise fanatic. He went back to school, eventually earning a degree as a Doctor of Chiropractic. What I admire most about him was his very early recognition of the dangers of processed foods and his lifelong campaign against them. His diet was nearly identical to the 'Paleo' diet that is gaining popularity today. And when you live to be 96, a 'lifelong campaign' constitutes quite a body of work.

He was a natural athlete. And here is where we differ. I am about as far from a natural athlete as it is possible to be. He maintained a regime of two hour workouts until his death. While I like the idea that 'you can do anything you put your mind to,' in practice, I find natural talent and ability is a strong predisposition. The media inundation of beautiful images gives us the fantasy that if we just use a deodorant, cosmetic, drive a particular car, or follow a particular diet or exercise regimen,

113

that we can transform ourselves into one of those images. I can think of no better way to sabotage a health regime than to compare myself to...well...anyone.

Now that we are approaching the final days of this 'reboot' I want to emphasize: this, like everything else in your life, is about being the honest, having integrity with yourself, and making the choices that will enhance your life. I spent many hours in the gym during the time that I worked at the YMCA, none of them wasted. Jane Fonda I was not. I am fairly certain that I tried every diet scam ever recommended, all of them espousing the exercise/ calorie restriction credo, and I am heavier now. Exercise, until the fifties, was thought to work against weight loss, and there is more and more evidence that gives this idea credence. In a recent documentary, 'Fed Up', it was stated that for a child to 'work off' a single cookie, he would need to ride a bicycle for an hour and fifteen minutes. Clearly, it has much more to do with what we are putting into our faces than with how we exercise.

That said, you have to exercise. What I have seen work, is to drop the term 'workout' from your vocabulary and use 'movement.' A workout is a trip to the gym, usually cardiovascular work, and a sense of self-righteousness; at least that is my experience. Movement is prioritizing moving throughout your waking hours. How that looks in my life is this: I spend a lot of time writing and on the computer. I have found that 40-45 minutes is my best work, and then my brain starts to spin its wheels. I set a timer (across the room, or in the kitchen so I have to get out of the chair to shut it up) and when it goes off, I make a quick note on where I am with the work, and where I would like to go next. The more often you do this, the more powerful it becomes as the rhythm sets up patterns in your brain. I get up, I try hard not to think, and I get a glass of water, hit the stationary bike hard for a few minutes, stretch or do 15 rapid upright rows with a 30# kettle bell (my current favorite.) There have to be at least a thousand sites with simple exercises that will get your heart rate jumping, which is the primary purpose. If you don't think you can make time to exercise, this is custom made for you. Once your eight hour day has been broken up with eight to ten of these intervals, you will have accrued an hour of exercise, stayed hydrated, and when you sit back at your desk, I guarantee that the fresh wash of oxygenated blood to your brain will often have clarified the next step in your work.

We prioritize efficiency in our culture, and busy-ness, or at least the appearance of being busy. Next time you empty the dishwasher, carry one dish at a time to the cabinet. When you pull laundry out of the dryer, hang it and take it to the closet, then go get another piece. During the commercial, do jumping jacks, although given the extended amount of commercials, we might be getting into workout range here.

The effect of even a small amount of movement is profound. As Jack Lallane grew older, he recognized the value of movement in the well-being of the elderly. I don't plan on pulling a boat from Alcatraz in handcuffs any time soon, but I also don't plan to go gently into that good night.

From an evolutionary perspective, I believe aging either transforms hormones or somehow changes our thought processes. The progeny of people who were willing and even happy to go out on the ice floes had more food and thus more chance of survival. A strong belief in an afterlife and a pretty miserable present life would certainly make that easier as well. But I have come to know that, at least for me, the antidote to an acceptance of aging, disability and death is movement. It is a powerful antidepressant, it swirls the blood through us to wash away the accrued sludge, and it feels good. I urge you to avoid the seductions of the recliner and remote, and to put on some music and dance.

Mussels have become very trendy, are still cheap, and supply a clean, mineral rich protein source. PEI are farmed mussels from Canada, grown in a clean and sustainable environment. Look for closed shells,

115

meaning they are still alive. A responsible fishmonger will sort through them for you. They need to be kept on ice until just before cooking.

Basic Steamed Mussels

½ pound mussels in the shell per person

Olive oil

Chopped garlic

Chopped parsley

Dry white wine

Put a large wide pan on the stove and heat the oil over medium heat. Add the garlic and cook just until you see it begin to brown, 30 seconds or so. Add an inch of white wine to the pan, then the mussels and quickly cover. In three minutes, check to see if they are opening. If not, check again every minute or so. Once most are opened, pour into a serving bowl and sprinkle with chopped parsley.

This is an excellent meal, fast and healthy. From here, once you own the technique, it is time to play. Add a can of tomatoes and a handful of shrimp with a few slices of sausage. Or go Asian, using lime juice, a splash of Vietnamese fish sauce or soy sauce, some minced ginger and a can of coconut milk instead of the wine. Maybe a piece of *kombu* in the cooking liquid? Add a salad and you have a meal.

My friend, Chef Billie Dixon has done a superlative job with the recipes he developed. They have been designed to teach you valuable kitchen skills, as well as introducing you to a new way of eating. I have been his sous chef and taster for many years, (a blessing I am grateful for daily), I can vouch that every one of the recipes is delicious. Like any new skill, cooking for yourself can be daunting, but is the very best investment you can make for your health. To beat the car metaphor to death, finally, you can be driving a Porsche Cayenne, just off the lot, but if you put bad fuel in you will run into trouble quickly. (And for the record, I married a mechanic, my son is a mechanic, and I know nothing about cars. I chose the Cayenne because it is very expensive and named after a food, so no need to send e-mails to tell me what a terrible investment it is. I just think it is pretty.)

Cooking for yourself and your family involves more than just standing by the stove and a few trips to the refrigerator. Shopping, planning, and often going to farmer's markets as well as groceries and big box stores plus researching and honing your skills can be intimidating. Let's look at some options. Racing to work, you forgo the bacon and eggs you could have fixed, or, given the time crunch, the shake you could have had in a jar in the fridge the night before, and hit the drive through instead. You need caffeine and a sugar lift would be a nice improvement on the morning, so you order a caramel coffee drink. Your 300 calories are made of 120 calories of fat. I am going out on a limb and guessing these are not organic grass fed, hormone and antibiotic free calories. No trans fats, but the USDA says that anything under .04 grams of this nasty stuff counts as zero. If anyone is keeping count. Your sugar jolt will be around 33 grams, which at 4.2 grams per teaspoon is nearly 8 teaspoons of sugar in a 16 ounce drink. There's fine start for the day.

But since you splurged on the drink, you get a muffin with fried egg whites and sausage. It says right on the menu that it only has 167 calories. 1180 grams of sodium (in the form of cheap commercial grade salt, not a mineral rich type like Himalayan Pink) doesn't count, since it isn't calories, and the 34 grams of carbohydrate (only three of which are, strictly speaking, sugar, but since they are from refined wheat flour, they will be higher on the glycemic index and metabolize more quickly) are most of the calories, in the bread. Since you sacrificed the egg yolk, where the heck did the 27 grams of fat come from? Some will be in the bun, of course, and you have to keep a lot of cheap fat on the grill so things don't stick… and oh yes, the 'mayonnaise' and 'pasteurized processed cheese like food' both have fat. Aren't you glad you passed on the egg yolk? That would have added 4.5 grams of pretty high quality fat, plus protein, Vitamins A & D, and some nice minerals. Oh wait. That would only happen if the chickens had been out in the sunshine eating a variety of bugs and grass and such. It might have been a good idea to forgo the yolk.

But you need to get a hash brown too. After all, you may have to work through lunch. 150 calories isn't bad. But 80 of those are from fat. And not fresh butter, trust me. It will be from overheated and overused 'vegetable oil' with a lot of soy oil. A sodium bump, again, not from Himalayan Pink salt with some other minerals, but from sodium and anti-caking chemicals. Beyond that, pretty much empty calories. And your taters had a long time to get homesick for Idaho, more than likely. They are often stored for months, if not years. But if there is no real food value to lose, what difference does it make?

Sure enough, you have to work through lunch, but the office sends out for food, and since you are still a little bilious from 'breakfast' you order a salad. Good for you. The greens were grown in the Central Valley of California a month ago. The person who planted it, cared for it and harvested it simply didn't have the time and certainly not the money to take care of his health. Field work with benefits is hard to find, much less a paid sick leave. Between that and your non-recyclable bowl sitting on your desk, at least ten other people handled your food. Sanitary facilities were likely to be minimal, but if you use enough chemicals in cleaning the lettuce, you can avoid a law suit. Remember, the appellation 'organic' means grown organically. We have yet to regulate processing. Many producers and restaurants use a nitrate soak to inhibit browning. It simply kills everything that could lead to oxidation, like enzymes, and guess what it does in your tummy? Yup. And the real treat is the dressing. Take a minute the next time you are in a grocery, and try to find a dressing without canola or soy oil. Then check the sugar and carbohydrate count.

The bottom line is this: If you want to regain your health, build your immune system and while you are at it, build a better greener world, you are going to have to find a system that you can trust to provide your food. Ideally, get it from the farmer who grew it. Not only does every cent stay in town, it stays with an entrepreneur who is working very hard to give me nutritious food. Follow the money. I would much rather see my dollars go for organic seed, a fair wage and benefits for workers, a new tractor and a spa day for everyone on the farm than for deceptive advertising and lobbyists.

Since 1992, which at this writing is 22 years, our government has urged us to use the USDA Food Pyramid as a nutritional guide. Be aware that this was formatted by lobbyists for the food industry and not by anyone with a priority of keeping us healthy. And we keep getting fatter and sicker. I know, a correlation isn't proof, but looking at it, 6-11 servings of grain as a base, let's say 6 pieces of bread. You get 120 calories, from each slice of bread, plus 23 grams of highly refined carbohydrates and 2 grams of sugar. That looks like 720 calories, 138 grams of carbohydrates and a nice fructose kick. In commercial bread, virtually all 'fortifications' are from cheap processed sources, so essentially, about a third of your calories for the day without taking in any nutrition to speak of. But there's more! It says between 6 and eleven servings so we are still on the extreme low end for consumption. Chinese food for

119

lunch? Add a cup and a half of rice to bring it to nine servings. That will bring it to 273 calories and 59 grams of carbohydrates, bringing the total to about 1000 calories, very damn few of which have any nutritional value. I am guessing that whatever there is has been pretty severely refined.

Next are fruits and vegetables. Potatoes, carrots and other high starch foods are included here. 5-6 servings of vegetables, and in our schools today, that can legally be pizza, now designated as a fruit because of its tomato sauce. 2-4 servings of fruit, and yes, fruit juice counts, although it is difficult to see a difference in the nutritional chart for orange juice and Coca Cola. All that Vitamin C? It evaporates quickly, and if a little is still in the juice, storage to preserve the 'freshness' can knock out the rest. Essentially, we are leaving a tiny amount of room for the top of the pyramid, the oils and fats, which I hope by now you have understood are crucial to health, particularly your brain and endocrine system. And the USDA sees no difference between highly refined rancid oils from soy and other seeds, and the vitamin and mineral rich fat found in grass-fed butter. Their only caution? 'Use sparingly'.

I am guessing the kitchen may hold a little more appeal now?

Convenience is a curse, often and highly seductive. This makes bread seem almost necessary, but there are other ways to make a meal portable. I make these ahead, then add the egg, broil for a couple of minutes and I am off! If you are grilling something, a few stuffed peppers off to the side to get some smokiness are wonderful, and they freeze well. Take one or two from the freezer to the fridge at night, and it should be thawed by morning. Crack an egg in, and add some leftover greens and maybe a little cheese if you are using dairy. You'll never miss your breakfast tacos.

Breakfast Sandwich to go

Three bell peppers, split vertically

1   pound cooked and seasoned beans or sausage, crumbled

6 eggs

Salsa

Put two Tablespoons of the crumbles sausage or beans into the pepper halves, crack in an egg, and slide under the broiler (about 4" away) for 3-5 minutes, depending on how you like your eggs. Top with salsa. If you are on the go, take them out underdone and wrap in foil, where they will continue to cook.

My favorite is black beans, egg, a spicy salsa and a little *cotija* cheese. Yummy, I mean yummy!

I hope you are still keeping up with the downloaded questions every evening; the information is priceless. (I know, nag, nag, nag, but it is my maternal gene coming out) Often a food intolerance is almost invisible, but puts tremendous strain on your system. I was certain that my nemesis, Diet Coke, was causing me little harm, if any. I mean all those people in the commercials are so beautiful and young and healthy, right? I had to avoid them 100% for over a month before I could really get an idea of how badly they made me feel. Sugar and grains and dairy all work the same way. It is supremely easy to tell myself: 'I AM listening to my body, and my body wants a freaking Diet Coke, RIGHT NOW!' But the difference between cravings and what your body actually needs is largely in the tone. If the desire for something is 'raising its voice' try to wait it out. If you feel hungry, but an apple doesn't sound good, you probably aren't hungry.

The truth is, we have lost variety in our diets. We are eating massive amounts of grains, most often in the form of HFCS. Most meals are accompanied by a large serving of grain, whether as a cereal for breakfast, a sandwich for lunch or pizza for dinner. Even if grains are not intrinsically a problem, the sudden increase in their consumption in any individual's diet crowds out the fruits and vegetables and proteins that our bodies need. Because grains are monocropped, and the manure is not returned to the soil, the vital minerals are gone. Many of these, like selenium and molybdenum are needed in tiny amounts, but are crucial to health and function. Because the last fifty years have flooded our food supply with refined carbohydrates and prepared foods and chemicals, for the sake of convenience, and because the food industry is a chronic and pathological source of misinformation and lies, our bodies have done what bodies do best- they have adapted. When we have more sugar in our blood stream because of overconsumption, our bodies struggle with it, and quickly learn to store it as fat, usually abdominal fat. As we get heavier, movement can become more difficult, and our metabolism slows.

Anyone who watches television could not be faulted if they believed that every physical problem is a pharmaceutical deficiency. We are 'out of balance.' But if there is any single skill that has moved us this far along the evolutionary trail, it is our bodies' ability to restore itself to balance. Famine, plague, disasters; we have beaten them all. Every one of us is a descendant of a lot of survivors. But what we are facing now, the pollution of our world and our food in particular looks like what may finally do us in. A creeping Ice Age is one thing to acclimate to over a few hundred years. But malnutrition in the midst of an overload of calories may do what the Bubonic Plague could never quite do.

And I started this chapter talking about cravings, only to pull out my old soapbox again on the evils of modern food. But these are two aspects of the same problem. The food industry has become a bloated science experiment to make cheap food so addictive (there's the craving part) that they can sell more and more every year. You have just spent a lot of time and effort avoiding this part of our culture. I'm requesting that in these last couple of days that you really look at how you feel. Do you feel strong and empowered? Disciplining yourself to make a number of very fundamental changes and accomplishing it for a month is a Big Deal. Not only have you gotten a lot of the accumulated muck out of your system, but you have also made a long term commitment and kept it. Bravo!

Does it feel like your brain is working differently? How exactly? If you meditate, even if you are just learning, how has that changed for you? Skin and hair changes? Pay attention as closely and in as much detail as you can and write it down. Are you happier? More creative? Like the diet that you will be developing in the coming days, what results you get from this program will be very individualized, but I really want you to write them down and be able to see what changes as you begin to reintroduce foods.

It can also be good to note what, if anything, you are craving. I don't think I made a single shake the first time I did this regime, without thinking that instead of using water to mix it, coffee would taste really, really good! Of course that was the first thing I reintroduced! Day 31, 6 a.m., I was standing by the coffee maker, relishing the gurgle, had my cup and discovered that I had become *much* more sensitive to caffeine. MUCH. This was a prime example to me of how accustomed I had become to managing the effects, because they were every day. It had become my normal.

I would suggest that, if you have eaten dairy in the past, you try a little early in the re-entry period. This can often result in a gut reaction, and occasionally in a skin reaction. Try just a small amount, and keep watch. If you are grain sensitive, it can have similar effects, but try adding only one grain at a time. Rice is the easiest to digest, and you may have kept it in your diet if you weren't trying to lose weight. Corn saturates our food supply, and I would try that next. Not a lovely corn on the cob, but something like cornbread which is made from the same sort of corn that HFCS is. Or have a soda. Read labels, to make sure that your reaction is to what you think it is rather than an additive. Wait a day between introductions, and observe. You have spent thirty days creating this powerful tool, so take advantage of it.

Lastly, food sensitivities don't have to be forever. If you avoid a food for several months, and eat a nutritionally dense diet, your body gets a rest from reacting to the food, and also gets the nutrition that it needs to manage the stress. A few months later, you <u>may</u> be able to add small amounts back into your meals on occasion.

Something that many people really miss is pizza. It has everything-convenience, cheap, refined flours and fats, chemical saturated meats and BPA canned tomatoes. What's not to like? It is possible to get the flavors of pizza without much of the downside though.

124

Eggplant Pizza

1 large eggplant, sliced in 1/2 " rounds

3-4 sliced tomatoes

¼ cup olive oil

1 Tablespoon balsamic vinegar

½ teaspoon oregano

Red pepper flakes to taste

Olives, cheese, peppers- whatever you like on a pizza

Preheat your oven to 450°. Toss the eggplant and tomato slices with the remaining ingredients to coat. Cover a sheet pan with parchment paper and lay the eggplant and tomatoes in a single layer on it. Bake for 15-20 minutes, turning once. Let cool, then arrange back on the parchment paper, overlapping the eggplant to form a solid base, and then topping with the tomatoes. Add whatever toppings you enjoy and broil until done.

Phase Three Chapter 29

I am sure you stayed up last night making notes. I am a chronic and compulsive journaler, and these last few years, I have added more observations than ever before about how my body is doing. It is amazing how much you can learn when you parallel disparate facts like how much and how well you slept, whether you took your supplements, any body changes, a food diary, and anything else you can think of. I am sure there is an app for it, but I am still doing it old school.

I am going to give you another fine tool that will be a tremendous help in reading your body. Back in the early fifties, Dr. Arthur Coca published a revolutionary book, called 'The Coca Pulse Test.' His wife had powerful reactions to foods, and they were having a great deal of difficulty determining what foods they were. Allergies can be tested for now, but these are only reactions to proteins, and as we know intolerances can be much more difficult to determine. He finally noticed that when his wife was about to have a reaction, her pulse would race. He went on to develop a four day regime, taking your pulse a total of 14 times during the day that may have saved his wife from a death by anaphylaxis. He went on to use it with his patients, with fine results and wrote the book. I found this to be an empowering practice and discovered a number of foods that I would never have thought I reacted to, because the symptoms were either subtle or something that I might have had on most days, like a slight headache.

If you have read 'A Nutritarian Notebook,' you already know about the 14 pulse, four day plan, but thanks to modern technology, I have come up with a much more efficient and accurate method. For the sake of convenience, you might want to get a heart rate monitor, which is not a bad thing to have anyway. Alternatively, there are apps that can measure and record your heart rate, but I have found them to be slightly less accurate. And counting your pulse, of course works too.

To proceed: Have a portion of the food you are going to test prepared, sit down comfortably, relax, and take a few deep breaths. Record you pulse rate, and if you are counting your heartbeats, go for a full minute. (Don't take fifteen seconds and multiply by four.) Now smell the food. I found this absolutely fascinating. By smelling a food, our bodies innately prepare to consume that exact thing. Take a few deep sniffs, and record your pulse again. If, at this point, you see a rise in your pulse of more than 4 beats per minute, your body is reacting to the food in a stressful way. You decide if you want to eat the food, and if so, hold it in your mouth for a full thirty seconds, and again, check your pulse. This is where the heart rate monitor earns its keep, as the numbers are immediate. If your pulse jumps more than 4 bpm from its resting rate, I would strongly suggest that you don't swallow the food!

The first time I did the four day test, was four years ago. I was quite stressed and ill, after several surgeries and the accompanying antibiotics and other medications. I was excruciatingly precise, and it seemed that I was reactive to everything I put in my mouth! This was a result of several things. I was so exhausted that I did react to practically anything. When I teach, I often use a glass bowl full of water and some small rocks as a visual aid, talking about stress und at the same time dropping the stones into the bowl. Pretty quickly, the water overflows, and I keep adding stones until someone says: 'Either quit adding the rocks or take some of them out!!' I was a big bowl full of rocks, teetering on each other and water cascading everywhere at that point in my life! Anything that even remotely stressed me was huge! (And can we see the evolution of the drama queen persona perhaps?)

It was quite an epiphany for me, and really got my attention. That was when I went back to school to certify as a Nutritional Therapist and began to reclaim my health. What a delight the whole thing has been... but I digress. I have used the pulse test off and on with a variety of foods. I find that restaurant food almost always shoots my pulse up, and I am guessing that MSG and unfermented soy products have a lot to

127

do with that. I really like the heart monitor method for restaurant use. Taking a bite of food, sniffing it, taking your pulse, tasting it and making notes ALWAYS makes you stand out. But gradually, as I have reduced the things in my life that kept me from thriving and added more movement and meditation and I prioritized my health above everything I have been able to eat small amounts of almost everything without getting myself all worked up. As I said in an earlier chapter, it is almost impossible to turn down a 4 year old's offer of her birthday cake, and now I don't have to.

It has been a long time with no dessert, barring a cheat day. Here is a very easy recipe, perfect for a summer afternoon.

Roasted Peach Ginger Ice Cream

1 pound peaches, peeled and sliced (3-4)

1 Tablespoon almond or coconut oil

1 can full fat coconut milk

1 teaspoon ground cinnamon

1 Tablespoon chopped crystallized ginger

1 oz. rum or brandy

Preheat oven to 400. Toss the peaches, oil and cinnamon together to coat. Line a sheet pan with parchment paper, and spread the peaches in a single layer. Roast for a total of 20 minutes, or until they begin to brown and caramelize. Let cool. Put into a blender with the coconut milk and booze and puree until smooth. When cooled completely, freeze according to ice cream maker's instructions, adding chopped ginger at the last. (The alcohol lowers the freezing point of the ice cream and helps prevent the formation of ice crystals. Optional.)

Phase Three, Chapter 30

You did it! And hopefully it was as much of an eye opener and a pleasure for you as it was for me. You'll be finishing up some of the supplements, and may find that you want to continue using some of them. The Biotics brand has been my choice for years, and unless the food based form is unstable, they make a tremendous effort to use organic food based sources, so that you absorb and get the benefit of their products. The Phase One supplements- Bromelain with CLA and the Beta tablets- are powerful supports for digestion.

The Beta TCP helps digest fats in particular. When our systems are overloaded and our livers become sluggish, adding the pancrelipase to our own bile supply can boost our ability to emulsify fats adequately to absorb them. And the beet extract is worth its weight in gold. When we eat a low fat diet, our gallbladders don't get the exercise they need. This small organ dumps bile onto the food leaving our stomach to break up the fats, but if there is not enough fat to stimulate it, then the bile thickens and can eventually create stones. Beets, whether fresh, raw, cooked, dried and powdered, act like paint thinner and increase the fluidity and movement of bile. Of course, hydration and getting some of those good fats into your diet, like grass fed butter, coconut oil and some nut oils is crucial too. And now that you have rebooted your palate as well, and are tasting things you never tasted before, look up the mayonnaise recipe and try it with macadamia oil...

Bromelain, from pineapple and papain from papayas are powerful proteolytic enzymes; they break down protein. If you have ever used a papaya based meat tenderizer, you have seen this in action. These are good to keep on hand to use with a largely protein meal. The morning you have steak and eggs would be a fine time to take a few, or anytime that you feel a little indigestion after a meal. These sorts of enzymes are also anti-inflammatory, particularly on an empty stomach.

129

Wobynzyme is perhaps the most widely known of the commercial enzyme tablets used for anti-inflammation, and is made of the same papain and bromelain. It has been used for many years in Europe, but has not been as popular in the United States although many people (me included) find it is a great help with muscle pain after exertion, and anecdotally, has sped my healing.

When I started writing, I had no real outline or idea of where it would go, and as I have heard other writers say, it developed a life of its own. The problem with writing something like this is that as I do the research and coalesce ideas, I learn so much, but once this is published, it doesn't change. I expect to keep learning and experimenting and tweaking until I die, and I am sure I will find there are many many things that I don't know at this moment, but I am hoping I have given you a start and empowered you to take responsibility for your health. Trusting other sources about what is happening within your body is necessary sometimes. But the more knowledge you have the better prepared you are for the challenge of staying healthy and happy in an increasingly more stressful, polluted and crazy world.

I must say, I feel a bit like I did when I took my son to his first day of kindergarten. Did I tell you everything you need to know to succeed and thrive? Did I tell you about candy and strangers, and that although the world is a little intimidating and frightening it is also beautiful? That a Cinnabon can be tempting, but that if you get away from it for a few weeks, a fresh warm strawberry that you pick yourself will stay in your memory, not your hips?

We are at a crossroads in America regarding food. I write letters every week to my Congress people about the food legislation that is benefitting the corporations and killing us. We can vote for a more responsive and functional Congress, and I pray that everyone does, but every dollar that we give to the prepared and refined food producers endorses them and every dollar that you take to a Farmer's Market and

130

hand over to the person who nurtured that plant or animal, watched it grow and flourish, responded to its needs and finally harvested it and put it in your hand is supporting so much! It calls for a return to real food, but also small local businesses and seasonal eating. It is creating a new sort of farmer who has an almost spiritual connection to his calling. It is slow food, cooked with love and relished with friends and family and with gratitude.

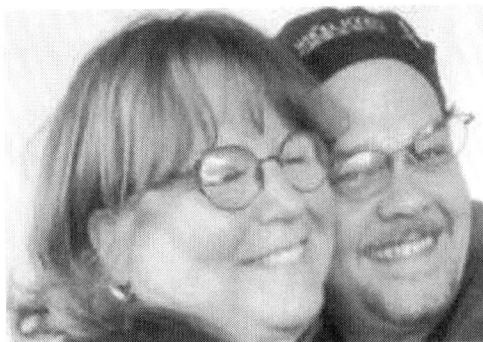

Billie Dixon and I have known each other for many years, if not many lifetimes. His culinary roots thrived deep in the Delta mud of Louisiana, and mine tumbleweeded through most of the Western United States, the last thirty plus years here in Austin. Billie studied Divinity (not the confection) and Cultural Anthropology at LSU, and twenty years earlier I studied Clinical Psychology at Arizona State. I married and raised a son and a stepdaughter and Billie birthed a restaurant, Crimson, near 6th Street in downtown Austin.

Food and family are the centers of our lives, and meals a sacrament. Growing up with Southern grandparents we learned from the cradle that food is love. And like love, there is a healthy variety and the less healthy sorts. When I went back to school, Billie was with me in spirit and a fine sounding board for my studies. The result has been my return to health and Billie losing well over a hundred pounds. We both are younger than when we met!

Billie and I have grieved and played and traveled together, but most of all we have laughed. A lot. It is a rare day that we don't connect. He is living and cooking in Asheville North Carolina, and I am still here in beloved Austin Texas. I love you Precious.

Foods to eliminate:

- **All grains except rice.** These are the most inflammatory foods and also the most common allergens. Gluten containing grains, especially wheat, rye, barley and oats, (aka BROW) can be especially damaging. You may not even know that you react to grains until you have a few weeks away from them to let your system relax and clear out. If you have blood sugar issues, eliminate rice as well.
- **Alcohol, caffeine, sodas, fruit juice and soy milk.** All of these are hard on the liver, and the whole idea is to give your liver a vacation.
- **Cold cuts, sausages, bacon, hot dogs, canned meats and shellfish.** Choose organically raised meats to avoid the antibiotics, hormones, nitrates and other additives typical of processed foods. Shellfish can contain mercury and other toxins, and are best to avoid for the time being.
- **Dairy.** This includes milk, cheese, butter and yogurt. These, like grains, are a common allergen. Avoiding them for a few weeks can be valuable in pinpointing food sensitivities. They can also be high in fat, and again, your liver is taking a well-earned rest.
- **All seed based oils, including peanut, margarine, shortening.** These processed oils are some of the most difficult for our bodies to process, as well as the most toxic. They require chemicals and heat which destroy any nutritional value. By using this program to cleanse your system you also have a chance to find alternatives to this toxic products and never use them again.
- **All refined sugars.** Like the oils, these refined carbohydrates are highly inflammatory. A great chance to eliminate them permanently.

o   **Any foods that you already know you are sensitive to.**

Approved Foods:

Eat as many of these as you like.

Vegetables: Alfalfa sprouts, arugula, avocado, bean sprouts, beets, broccoli, brussels sprouts, cabbage, carrots, cauliflower, celery, collards, cucumber, garlic, kale, lettuce, mushrooms, mustard greens, olives, onions, radish, snow peas, spinach, string beans, sweet potatoes, squash, tomatoes (fresh only, no canned).

Fruits: Berries, melons, apples, bananas, citrus, kiwi, figs, grapes, mangoes, pears and plums.

Fats: Almonds, cashews, coconut oil, olive oil, pecans, tahini, walnuts.

Protein: (organic strongly preferred) Beef, black beans, chicken, cod, duck, free range eggs, garbanzos, lamb, lentils, pinto beans, red beans, red snapper, salmon, shrimp, tuna and turkey.

Dairy Alternatives: Rice milk, coconut milk, hemp milk.

Starch: Rice, rice crackers, rice pasta.

Beverages: Lots of water in small increments throughout the day. Green tea.

Sweeteners: Honey, maple syrup

Dressings: Olive oil, nut oils (walnut, almond, pecan and sesame) should be kept in moderation. They can be used with unpasteurized vinegar or citrus juice, and any fresh or dried herbs. Salt and pepper are fine. Do avoid balsamic vinegars, as they contain fructose.

Water: 1 liter or more on waking, before eating. Add lemon juice if

134

desired.

As you can see, there is a lot of variety allowed, and infinite possibilities.

Date:

I woke at_____

I slept 1 2 3 4 5 6 7 8 9 10 hours

I dreamed about:

I feel rested   y n

I am grateful for:

I took my morning supplements y n

My bathroom experience:

For breakfast I had:

I felt optimistic about the day   1 2 3 4 5 6 7 8 9 10

My exercise plan for the day is:

135

My exercise for the day ended up being:

For lunch I had:

I remembered to:

I meditated today   y   n

How long:

I laughed today at:

For dinner I had:

I took my evening supplements   y   n

The best thing I did for my health today was:

The worst thing I did for my health today was:

I thanked   _____

for_____

What is working well for me today?

136